Tutorials in Surgery 2

Tutorials in Surgery 2

F G Smiddy, MD, ChM, FRCS

*Senior Clinical Lecturer in Surgery,
University of Leeds.*

*Member of the Court of Examiners of the
Royal College of Surgeons, England.*

*Examiner in Pathology to the College of
Surgeons, England.*

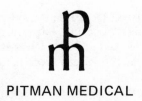

PITMAN MEDICAL

First published 1979

Catalogue Number 21 3444 81

Pitman Medical Publishing Co Ltd
P O Box 7, Tunbridge Wells,
Kent, TN1 1XH, England

Associated Companies

UNITED KINGDOM
Pitman Publishing Ltd, London
Focal Press Ltd, London

CANADA
Copp Clark Pitman, Toronto

USA
Fearon Pitman Publishers Inc, San Francisco
Focal Press Inc, New York

AUSTRALIA
Pitman Publishing Pty Ltd, Melbourne

NEW ZEALAND
Pitman Publishing NZ Ltd, Wellington

British Library Cataloguing in Publication Data

Smiddy, Francis Geoffrey
Tutorials in surgery.
2.
1. Surgery
I. Title
617   RD31

ISBN: 0 272 79545 3

Set in 10 on 11 pt IBM Press Roman by
Gatehouse Wood Ltd, Edenbridge, Kent
Printed and bound in Great Britain
at The Pitman Press, Bath

Contents

Preface

This second volume of surgical tutorials is designed, like its predecessor, to be of use to pre- and postgraduate students who are studying for their final examinations. The format of Tutorials 1 has been followed as closely as possible, although I have attempted to avoid the criticism of the first volume made by Professor Harold Ellis that a diagram here and there amid the text might be of help. In places, therefore, in which they seem appropriate these have been included.

It has given me great pleasure to write this volume since the majority of the work was done while I was suffering from an injury that made all activities, other than reading and writing, impossible. I hope it gives as much pleasure to the reader and also that it is of as great an educational value to the reader as it was to the writer.

F.G. Smiddy
January, 1979

To my new family

Paul and Katy Smiddy

Acknowledgements

As with all books this one was not written without considerable assistance. It gives me great pleasure to acknowledge the efforts of Elaine Clutterbuck, Joan Desborough, Chantel Meystre, Anna Wright, M. Green, J.P. Watson, J.J. Amor, J.A. Clarke and J.G.H. Bottomley, all members of one of my 'firms', who did a considerable amount of preliminary work on some of the topics discussed in this volume.

I am also grateful to Dr L.A.D. Tovey, Director of the Leeds Regional Blood Transfusion Service, for his help on the section devoted to haemophilia, and to Dr R. Collins, Senior Lecturer in Mathematics at the University of Salford, who was able to explain the nuances of Bayes's theorem in a manner totally understandable to the non-mathematically-minded surgeon.

Lastly, as ever, I am grateful for the devotion shown by Mrs P. Docherty who has repeatedly retyped the script as this became necessary until finally order came out of chaos.

1 General Principles

1.1 CARCINOGENIC AGENTS

Definition. A carcinogen is an agent which, in a given population, significantly increases the yield of malignant neoplasms or causes neoplasms that otherwise would not develop to do so. A malignant neoplasm may be defined as an abnormal mass of cells the growth of which exceeds and is unco-ordinated with that of normal tissue and which persists in the same excessive manner after the cessation of the stimulus that wrought the change. The essential attribute of a malignant tumour is its ability to invade the tissues of the host.

In 1938, Shear introduced the term cocarcinogen to describe substances which, of themselves, would not produce cancer, but when combined with a subcarcinogenic dose of a solitary carcinogen produce a neoplasm. In such systems the solitary carcinogen may be an alkylating agent or an aromatic hydrocarbon, often termed 'the tumour initiator', whereas the cocarcinogen may be croton oil, tobacco smoke, phenols, etc. The cocarcinogen is often known as the tumour promoter. The carcinogenic agents are divisible into three major groups—

1 Ionising irradiation   2 Viruses   3 Chemical agents.

Of greatest importance at the present time are the chemical agents because—

(*a*)   exposure to ionising irradiation is nowadays under very strict control, and

(*b*)   whereas members of groups 1 and 3 have been directly incriminated in the production of human cancer no such claim can be made for the viruses.

In addition to these exogenous forms of stimuli that lead to cancer it is also apparent that, in the human, certain genetic diseases are associated with malignancy. In some cases the primary defect is immunological, e.g. a high

1

incidence of leukaemia and lymphoreticuloses are found in congenital agammaglobulinaemia, which is X-linked. In other conditions, no such immunological defect exists, e.g. in Garner's syndrome, which is an autosomal dominant disease associated with a high incidence of carcinoma of the colon and endocrine tumours.

Ionising irradiation

The mechanisms of cancer induction by radiation remains obscure. In terms of potency and specificity, radiation does not compare with many other cancer-inducing agents and, indeed, it is much more effective as a cytotoxic agent than as a carcinogenetic agent. Nevertheless, in the experimental animal, the implantation of a radioactive source emitting α or β rays will produce neoplasia, the type varying according to the tissue into which the implant is made. In mice and rats, partial body irradiation produces cancers or sarcomata within ten to twenty-four months. In general, irradiation is followed by cancer only if the dose is severe enough to cause tissue damage. The effect of irradiation may be local, with the production of tumours in the immediate vicinity of the source, or remote, when tumours are induced in organs not directly irradiated. In the experimental animal, bone-seeking isotopes such as ^{32}P, ^{90}Sr, ^{226}Ra or ^{239}P will all produce tumours if given in large enough doses. A comparison of the effectiveness of the different isotopes suggests that α emissions are the important factor, and proximity to osteogenic tissue.

Whole body irradiation in animals will give rise to leukaemia, which may be regarded as a cancer of the bone marrow cells. In some mice the induction of leukaemia appears to depend on the liberation of a viral agent, which is then believed to initiate the change.

In man, the most well-documented human cases of irradiation induced leukaemia are those from the atomic explosions of Hiroshima and Nagasaki in which it was found that the incidence of leukaemia was related to the dose of radiation received and the time that elapsed following exposure. The dose could be measured by knowing the distance of the victim from the hypocentre. As this distance increased, the incidence of leukaemia fell; at 1000 m the case incidence was $7000/10^6$, whereas at 2500 m the incidence had fallen dramatically to $63/10^6$.

Other examples of irradiation-producing human cancers are the high incidence of skin cancers that once were common in the early radiologists, the incidence of leukaemia in patients irradiated for the treatment of ankylosing spondylitis, and the high incidence of thyroid cancers that followed the treatment of children for 'supposed' thymic enlargement by external irradiation of the superior mediastinum.

One notorious case of industrial irradiation was found in the watch industry in which women were employed to paint luminous watch dials. The paint used contained a mixture of radium and mesothorium; to the latter is attributed the local necrosis of the jaws that used to follow employment in this industry, and to the former the development of anaemia and osteogenic sarcoma. The effect was due to the β particle irradiation, and the incidence of tumour formation was of the order of 20 per cent after a latent period of between 19 and 31 years.

Another form of irradiation is that of exposure to excessive ultraviolet light. In humans, the critical part of the spectrum lies between 290 and 330 nm Å. Australian farmers characteristically develop keratotic papillomata on the face and hands which later develop into multiple squamous or basal cell carcinomata.

A similar but much more extreme sensitivity to ultraviolet light is observed in patients suffering from xeroderma pigmentosum in whom DNA once injured by u.v. cannot be repaired.

Viral agents

The oncogenic viruses are largely of interest to the experimental cancer worker. The first such virus was discovered in 1908 when the Shope rabbit papilloma was described. The Shope rabbit, known as the 'wild cotton-tail', is found in Kansas and Iowa. This rabbit develops large tumours on the skin of the abdomen, neck and shoulder, which appear as horny warts. The disease can be transmitted by rubbing the scarified skin with a filtrate of the tumour but it cannot be transmitted by injecting the extract into muscles or internal organs.

A second virus of experimental importance is the Rous chicken sarcoma virus. This virus is a spherical particle about 75 nm in size which is visible by electron microscopy within the cytoplasm but not in the nucleus of affected cells.

Other animal viruses extensively investigated include the herpes virus which in chickens induces lymphomatous disease, commonly called Marek's disease after the Hungarian pathologist who described the condition in 1907. This condition led to huge losses in the poultry industry which, in turn, led to intensive research and to the isolation of the responsible virus and, finally, the production of live virus vaccines either based on tissue culture attenuated or antigenically related herpes virus derived from the turkey.

Despite investigation the viral products required to effect and maintain the cellular changes resulting in neoplastic growth are unknown.

In man, the cancers under the most intensive investigation in relation to a possible viral aetiology are the lymphomas, mammary cancer, and certain sarcomas.

Much effort has been devoted to elucidate the role of the Epstein Barr herpes virus in Burkitt's lymphoma. The virus was first isolated from Burkitt's lymphoma in 1964. The disease itself has certain attributes all of which suggest the importance of environmental factors. These include—

(*a*) a geographical area of incidence limited by the 60°F isotherm within sub-Saharan Africa, Papua and New Guinea;

(*b*) seasonal variations;

(*c*) a high incidence between 2 and 14 years with a peak incidence at nine years of age.

However, this virus is also found in association with nasopharyngeal carcinoma, and EBV antibodies are also found in the benign self-limiting disease of infectious mononucleosis. The almost universal distribution of the virus somewhat detracts from its potential importance as the sole aetiological factor in Burkitt's lymphoma. Possibly the only children to develop Burkitt's lymphoma are those who do not possess a high enough antibody titre.

Slightly greater specificity is claimed for the Bittner milk factor which is a thermolabile agent in two forms, an intracytoplasmic particle 65 nm in diameter and an extracytoplasmic particle 105 nm in diameter. Virus particles identical with the Bittner factor have been found in human breast cancer cells and also in Parsee female breast tissue. The Parsees have an exceptionally high incidence of breast cancer which coincides with a very high incidence of particles.

Chemical carcinogens

The first experimental chemically induced tumour of the skin was produced by Yamagiwa and Ichikawa, in 1915, when they painted rabbits' ears with coal tar and produced squamous epithelioma. Since then it has been established that the organic chemical agents capable of producing experimental cancers can be divided into three groups.

Group 1   Polycyclic hydrocarbon

In 1775, Percival Pott described the possible connection between occupation and cancer when he described chimney sweep's cancer of the scrotum. He pointed out that exposure to soot began in infancy and was followed in adolescence by tumour formation. Thereafter, a variety of occupational tumours were described: the scrotal cancers of copper and tin workers due to exposure to arsenic and, in 1875, the shale-oil cancers found on the scrotum, hands and arms of primary producers and users.

In 1931, Kennaway isolated 1,2,5,6-dibenzanthracene, the first pure chemical to have carcinogenic properties, and later, methylcholanthrene and 3,4-benzpyrene were also shown to be powerful carcinogens producing papillomas and carcinomas when applied to the skin, and sarcomas when subcutaneously administered. The carcinogenic polycyclic hydrocarbons are considered to be initiators, see above, producing an irreversible change in the cells of the target organ following a single exposure. The development of tumours from such cells, i.e. promotion, may be achieved either by the application of further hydrocarbon or a non-carcinogenic material such as croton oil, the active agents of which are long chain fatty acid esters of the complex terpene.

4

The polycyclic hydrocarbons are found in pitch, tar, car exhaust fumes, and the condensate of tabacco smoke. It is, therefore, likely that the lungs and bronchi are exposed to benzpyrene and other hydrocarbons. Possibly, the difference in incidence of lung cancer between the USA and England is related to the coal tar products used for asphalting the roads in the latter country, for the amount of smoking appears to be the same but the incidence of cancer of the bronchus is higher.

Group 2   Aromatic amines

The main health hazard of these chemicals in man is cancer of the urothelial tract, principally affecting the urinary bladder. There are eight main occupational groups in which there is a raised incidence of bladder cancer. These include the chemical and dyestuff industries, pigment and paint manufacturers, rubber workers, and workers in the tar and pitch industries. The amines active in man include 2-napthylamine, benzidine, fuchsin, auramine and zenylamine. The relationship between occupation and exposure to the chemicals was proven on statistical grounds when it was found that workers in certain industries developed bladder cancer nearly fifteen years earlier than the general population.

However, 2-napthylamine does not induce tumours when implanted in the mouse bladder or instilled into the bladder of dogs. The carcinogenic agent is a metabolite 2-amino-l-napthol which is an intermediary product found in the liver. Once produced, this is detoxicated by conjugation with glucuronic acid but in man and dogs the bladder excretes a β-glucuronidase which splits this compound and liberates the carcinogen.

Group 3   Azo compounds

These include scarlet red and butter yellow, the active principle in the latter being 4-dimethylamino azo benzine, a compound that leads to the development of liver tumours in rats after being bound to the protein in the hepatocyte. Commercially, the azo compounds are used as colouring materials in prepared foods.

In addition to the organic compounds already described, far simpler chemical compounds can induce cancer in man, examples being the increased incidence of lung and nasal cancer found in nickel workers and the development of cancer in workers exposed to asbestos dust.

1.2   BIOLOGICAL ASPECTS OF TUMOUR GROWTH

Introduction. The overall size of a normal fully grown individual remains relatively constant. This does not mean that cellular division has ceased, although it is certainly true for the central nervous system which once having reached maturity slowly atrophies, a change particularly evident in the basal ganglia which, if the atrophy is severe, causes Parkinson's disease, and in the cerebrum, causes senile dementia. At the opposite end of the spectrum are the cells of the skin, the mucous membrane of the gastrointestinal tract and the haemopoietic system in all of which division occurs in order to replace effete cells. The rate of cellular division has been most thoroughly quantified in the haemopoietic system because the life span of an erythrocyte can be readily determined following labelling with radioactive chromium. Such methods show that the half-life of the erythrocyte is about 60 days and if the curve for loss of radioactivity is suitably corrected it is found to be almost linear, falling to zero in about 120 days. Since the average red cell count is 5×10^{12} litre and the average blood volume for a man of 70 kg body weight is 5 litres it can be calculated that the number of red cells replaced daily by the normal marrow is approximately 2×10^9. Despite this enormous number, control is maintained so that the count does not fall and lead to anaemia or rise to produce the equally undesirable condition of polycythaemia. Similarly, the time required for the turnover of the mucosal cells of the gastrointestinal tract has been established by the use of tritiated thymidine which is incorporated into the desoxyribonucleic acid of their nuclei, thus enabling the cells to be traced by serial biopsy. This type of investigation has shown that in the stomach and duodenum, the turnover time is approximately two days, in the jejunum four days, and in the rectum seven days.

The factors that control these normal processes of cell division remain uncertain although it is relatively obvious that, *ab initio*, growth must depend upon some inherent property of the fertilised ovum. In the child, the presence of growth hormone is essential since it is responsible for the normal rate of protein synthesis and fat metabolism. Deficiency of growth hormone alone leads to one type of dwarfism 'sexual ateliotic' in which the individual remains short but matures sexually. At the cellular level it has been shown that cells of like structure, e.g. embryonic kidney cells, aggregate together in tissue culture even though initially separated. Having come into contact with one another the ability of such cells to divide is limited, a limitation believed to be due to contact, one cell with another. Such contact inhibition can, however, be altered by treating the cell with proteolytic enzymes, and it has been assumed that this phenomenon must be absent in the malignant cell. The affinity of cells for their own kind must be of great importance in the development of multicellular animals but even so, not all groups of cells behave in the same manner, blood cells for example do not exhibit adhesiveness nor to any great extent do malignant cells.

Cellular division

The most important feature in the division of a single cell is mitosis or the division of the cell nucleus into two, a process necessary to conserve the

6

specific number of chromosomes in each cell, which in man is 46. Four stages are recognised—

1 The prophase during which the chromosomes become visible within the nucleus as long thin filaments which progressively shorten and thicken. At this stage each chromosome has already split into its two daughter chromosomes, the chromatids, although each pair is held together by the centromere. At the same time, the cytoplasmic body, known as the centriole, divides to produce two centrioles which move to opposite poles of the cell and it is from these bodies that the protein fibres known as the spindle radiate. As this phase ends the nuclear membrane, which is composed of two laminae each about 7.5 nm in width, disappears.

2 The metaphase. During this phase the microtubules, known as the spindle, are formed and radiate from the centrioles situated at the opposite poles of the cell. The chromosomes arrange themselves in the equatorial plane of the cell lying across the developing spindle and attached to it by their centromeres forming the equatorial plate.

3 The anaphase. At this stage the two chromatids separate following a longitudinal division of the centromere. The spindle fibres now appear to contract, pulling the chromatids, which have become the chromosomes of the two daughter nuclei, towards the opposite poles of the cell. Once this has been accomplished a cleavage furrow appears in the cell membrane indicating the beginning of cellular division.

4 The telophase, in which the chromosomes elongate and disappear as the new nuclear membrane forms and the spindle disappears. At this point cellular division is completed and the cell enters the resting phase, which is also known as the interphase, during which the chromosomes cannot be detected inside the nucleus as discrete structures by a light microscope although a few condensations of DNA can be recognised, one of which is the sex chromatin, the Barr body.

The interphase is normally divided into three—

(*a*)   the G1 phase, in which ribonucleic acid (RNA) synthesis occurs associated with growth of the cell, but no desoxyribonucleic acid (DNA) is formed;

(*b*)   S phase, in which the DNA replicates;

(*c*)   G2 phase, in which further growth occurs.

Biochemistry of cellular division

The two most important constituents of the cell in respect of cellular division, are the nucleic acids. These are made up of many thousands of units known as nucleotides, each of which consists of three further subunits, a phosphate group, a pentose sugar and a nitrogen-containing base. In DNA the sugar component is desoxyribose whereas in RNA it is ribose.

DNA contains four different nitrogenous bases, the pyrimidines, cytosine, thymine and the purines, adenine and guanine. RNA also has four bases but thymine is replaced by a different pyrimidine, uracil.

The sugar and phosphate groups form alternate links in the chain and the nitrogenous bases are attached to the sugar units at right angles. The DNA complex exists as two chains which are twisted into a helix and wound around one another in a spiral fashion, the two opposing spirals linked together by hydrogen bonds which connect the nitrogenous bases projecting into the space between the strands.

The nature of the hydrogen bonds joining these base pairs is highly specific so that adenine unites with thymine and guanine with cytosine. As a result of this arrangement, if the sequence of bases on one chain is known, those on the other can be deduced.

The structure of the DNA molecule ensures that when the cell divides the sequence of bases which constitute the genetic code will be carried to the next generation so that the new chromosomes will be identical with the old. Replication or division of the RNA strand results from the breaking of the hydrogen bonds, which thus releases the base pairs. Such unpaired bases would be free to pick up other bases from their surroundings but because of the specific nature of the hydrogen bonds each can only join with one of the four available. Once the bases are paired, linking enzymes bring the sugar and phosphate groups together to form the new DNA strand.

Cell cycle of the normal cell

It was once considered that DNA synthesis was a continuous process but the use of radioactive thymidine has shown that it is phasic. During the two resting phases known as G1 and G2 respectively, the DNA content of the cell remains static, but sandwiched between these is the S or synthetic phase during which the DNA content of the cell doubles. Following phase G2 mitosis occurs. However, it has been shown that some cells with a capacity to divide pass ino a resting phase of variable length known as the Go phase from which they may, following a suitable stimulus, once more pass into the G1 phase in preparation for division.

The percentage of cells in the Go phase in the bone marrow has been variously estimated at between 20 and 50 per cent of the whole cellular population. The common stimulus which promotes division of this particular cellular population is haemorrhage. The fraction of cells that are actively dividing, the growth fraction, varies in different tissues but in 'tumours' it is estimated that as many as 90 per cent of the total population of tumour cells may be in the Go phase. Further, in a malignant tumour, the cell population is very heterogenous, consisting of some cells that are capable of an infinite number of divisions until death of the host occurs, and others that are capable of only four or five divisions before this particular 'clone' of cells dies out.

In vitro studies have shown that the various phases in the cell cycle vary a great deal in duration. The G1 phase may last up to 30 hours whereas the synthetic phase is normally between 6 and 8 hours, the G2 phase between 2 and 4 hours, and mitosis is usually accomplished in 1 hour.

Cell cycle of the malignant cell

The cell cycle of a malignant cell is remarkably similar to that of a normal cell, the total duration of the cycle varying between 40 and 80 hours. The reason a tumour grows is because any division of a cancerous cell increases the total cellular population whereas a normal cell divides only to replace a cell which has been lost so that the overall population remains constant.

However, the growth of a tumour does not follow the pattern that would result from the repeated division of a single stem cell; if this were so, the tumour would double in size with each cellular division. This is not so; depending on the tissue studied, the doubling time of a tumour may vary between 4 and 500 days, being most rapid for the leukaemias and slowest for the solid cell carcinomata.

This variation in doubling time is caused by a number of factors—

(*a*) Loss of cells from the surface of a tumour. This is a particularly important factor when considering tumours of the gastrointestinal and urinary tracts which are continuously exfoliating, hence the technique of exfoliative cytology.

(*b*) Tumour necrosis. In all tumours the vascular supply is not only abnormal, but in order to grow and undergo mitosis the malignant cell, like the fibroblast, also requires a certain minimum concentration of oxygen and, therefore, a certain proximity to their blood supply. Experimentally it can be shown that the cell cycle time, i.e. the time required for division, remains the same in hypoxic conditions as in a well-oxygenated environment *but* the dividing fraction of cells gradually diminishes as the anoxia increases.

(*c*) Many tumour cells are so abnormal that they can divide only through a few generations before finally dying.

(*d*) Metastasisation. A certain percentage of tumour cells will be lost as they are washed away from the primary site either via the blood stream or the lymphatics.

(*e*) Host resistance. The gradually increasing importance of cellular immunity in the host's defence against neoplastic cells is becoming increasingly recognised. It has been suggested that immunological surveillance by an immunologically competent host is capable of the total destruction of small tumours. It is also an undisputed fact that in patients in whom this system is damaged either by drugs, by radiotherapy, or as the result of immunodeficiency disease there is an increase in the incidence of tumours, particularly of the lymphoid system. There is also some evidence, for example, that the histological reaction in the lymph nodes in proximity to a carcinoma of the breast can be correlated with survival rate.

The number of cells lost to a tumour in the various ways described may result in the loss of as many as 99 per cent of all those produced. Nevertheless, this still results in tumour growth since the cell population in a given tissue is increased.

In summary, therefore, the rate of tumour growth is dependent upon—

(a) the time taken for the tumour cells to divide;
(b) the fraction of cells actually dividing;
(c) the loss of cells from the developing tumour.

It is this combination that determines the doubling time. In human leukaemias, growth is exponential in that there is a proportional increase in tumour cells per unit of time, but this does not apply to the majority of solid tumours which are those of greatest interest to the surgeon.

So far as the clinician is concerned a cancer in a superficial organ such as the breast is rarely detected before it has doubled in size approximately 30 times thereby producing a palpable mass approximately 1 cm in diameter and weighing between 1 and 2 g. The following 10 to 14 doublings, assuming uninterrupted growth is allowed to continue, will result in a mass approximately 1 kg in weight by which time death has usually occurred. Obviously the duration of life is intimately related to the tissue within which the tumour is growing. A patient suffering from a carcinoma of the colon in whom hepatic metastases are already recognisable at the time of the initial operation may live for as long as three years, whereas the physiological consequences of increasing intracranial pressure produces death in a short time in patient's suffering from primary or metastatic malignant disease of the brain

1.3 CYTOTOXIC AGENTS, THEIR EFFECTS ON NORMAL AND TUMOUR TISSUES

1 Alkylating agents

This group includes such compounds as thiotepa, phenylalanine mustard, chlorambucil, cyclophosphamide, bisulphan, and there are many others. The fundamental observation, which led to the use of these agents for the treatment of cancer, was that nitrogen mustard, first used as a war gas, had an antimitotic potential.

The alkylating agents exert their cytotoxic effect by developing cross linkages or bridges between opposite guanine bases, thus binding the DNA strands together and preventing them from separating at the time of replication. Where separation is still able to occur the alkylating agents attach themselves to the free guanine bases so preventing them from acting as templates for the formation of new DNA.

2 Antimetabolites

This group includes methotrexate, 5-mercaptopurine, 5-fluorouracil and cytarabine hydrochloride.

The action of the antimetabolites results from the structural similarity which exists between them and the normal cellular metabolites required for protein synthesis, a similarity well illustrated by that which exists between methotrexate and the vitamin folic acid.

Methotrexate is a folic acid antagonist because it has a much greater affinity for the enzyme dihydrofolate reductase than folic acid. Once methotrexate combines with this enzyme the combination is inseparable and as a result folinic acid, the essential co-enzyme into which folic acid is converted, is no longer formed. In the absence of the co-enzyme the synthesis of purines and pyrimidines ceases. In a similar manner 5-fluorouracil, which is a pyrimidine in which a fluorine atom is substituted for a hydrogen atom, probably blocks the enzyme thymidilate synthetase. This is essential to pyrimidine synthesis, deficiency inhibiting the formation of thymine and cytosine and so preventing DNA replication.

3 Vinca alkaloids

This group consists of vincristine and vinblastine. The vinca alkaloids arrest cell division at the metaphase, probably by interfering with spindle formation so that the chromatids cannot be properly paired, and mitosis ceases.

4 Antimitotic antibiotics

This group contains actinomycin D, daunorubicin and bleomycin. They act by forming irreversible complexes with single strands of the DNA molecule inserting themselves between the bases and attaching themselves by hydrogen bonds to the guanine moiety of the DNA chain, thus preventing DNA synthesis.

5 Nitrosoureas

A group which includes carmustine, lomustine, semustine and 1-methyl-2-nitrourea. These compounds act in a similar manner to the alkylating agents and in addition inhibit mitosis by blocking the enzymes responsible for purine synthesis and the incorporation of purine into DNA. Unlike many antitumour agents the nitrosoureas are lipid soluble and are, therefore, able to pass through the blood brain barrier.

6 Miscellaneous group

This includes procarbazine, hydroxycarbamide, hexamethylmelanine and asparaginase. The latter compound is of particular interest because theoretically it exploits one of the few biochemical differences that exist between normal and malignant cells. Asparagine is an amino acid essential to human cells. Unlike normal cells, however, malignant cells are unable to synthesise it and as a result have to rely on the supply of this amino acid from the general pool.

Asparaginase is an enzyme that splits asparagine into aspartic acid and ammonia. Theoretically, therefore, if the body is flooded with this enzyme the body pool of free asparagine should fall and the malignant cell should be denied an essential nutrient. Unfortunately, in practice the efficacy of this drug has not lived up to its theoretical promise. In a similar fashion the drug phenylalanine mustard has also been a disappointment. Theoretically, the latter drug should have been extremely effective in the treatment of malignant melanoma because melanin-producing cells require phenylalanine in order to produce pigment. Using phenylalanine mustard, therefore, it might have been expected that the alkylating agent would have been specifically taken into the melanoma cell in much higher concentration than into normal cells, thus producing differentially higher concentrations of the alkylating agent.

ALTERNATIVE CLASSIFICATION OF THE CYTOTOXIC AGENTS

This has been based on the point in the cell cycle at which the drug exerts its effect, for example, nitrogen mustard resembles the action of X-rays in that cells in all stages of division are destroyed. The remaining agents have been divided into the Cell Cycle Stage Specific Group (CCSS). This includes 6-mercaptopurine and methotrexate which act only during the period of DNA synthesis (the S phase) and the Cell Cycle Non Specific Group (CCNS). This group includes 5-fluorouracil, actinomycin and cyclophosphamide which although having little effect on cells in the resting (Go) phase, kill cells at all other stages with equal effectiveness. Although such a classification should have therapeutic implications, in practice these cannot yet be exploited.

Other methods, at present only of theoretical interest, by which it has been suggested malignant disease may be controlled, are—

1 by the development of drugs capable of affecting tumour angiogenesis;
2 by the prevention of cellular implantation, on which the successful development of metastases depends;
3 by the development of cytostatic agents capable of arresting cellular development without necessarily destroying them;
4 by increasing the specificity of the agent so that it is taken up in higher concentration by the tumour cell than by the normal cells. An early example of this already quoted was the introduction of phenylalanine mustard.

EFFECTS OF CYTOTOXIC AGENTS ON NORMAL TISSUES

Cytotoxic agents produce toxic effects on normal tissues because there is little to distinguish normal and malignant cells. The result is that cells proliferating during the normal course of physiological repair or replacement may be damaged. This harmful effect is greatest on rapidly dividing tissues and it is the resultant damage to these tissues that limits the usefulness of these drugs. However, all drugs do not produce to the same degree the toxic changes that have been described.

Specific effects

The rapidly dividing tissues that suffer such harmful effects from cytotoxic agents include the bone marrow, the lining cells of the gastrointestinal tract and the skin.

1 The bone marrow is especially vulnerable since the doubling time of the stem cells of the bone marrow is only 15 to 20 hours compared with a tumour system in which the doubling time may be as long as 500 days. The first noticeable toxic effect is on the white cells the life span of which is only 4 to 5 days. Later, the number of platelets with a life span of approximately ten days falls, and lastly, anaemia develops, usually within 8 weeks, if a drug is being given continuously.

In some patients, total marrow failure may occur and the failure may not be reversible.

2 In the gut, mitosis ceases in the stem cells which lie in the crypts of Lieberkühn, with the result that the mucosa of the small bowel rapidly degenerates as the villi swell and become distorted.

These changes are accompanied by gross exudation and so great a decrease in the resistance of the gut to bacterial invasion that septicaemia may occur.

3 The commonest toxic change involving the skin is the suppression of hair growth, leading to alopecia. This is always reversible although the new hairs may be of different texture from the old.

In addition to these common effects the surgeon should also remember—

(*a*) that the embryo is a mass of rapidly dividing cells and that cytotoxic agents given in the first trimester are a potent cause of fetal abnormality; and

(*b*) that the lymphoid system, which is responsible for the production of the immunoglobulins and immunologically competent lymphocytes may also be damaged. This has two possible adverse effects; first, a failure to form antibodies and, hence, an increased susceptibility to infection, a susceptibility increased by the concomitant decrease in the granulocyte population; and secondly, a potential loss of those immune mechanisms helping to suppress tumour growth.

13

Effect of a cytotoxic agent on the tumour cell

When initially introduced, single cytotoxic agents were most commonly used over long periods in doses that caused minimal signs of toxicity. This technique was in accord with the then accepted principle that tumours increased in size because of the more rapid division of their cell population than normal tissues. Approximately twenty years ago combination therapy was introduced in which two or more drugs, each with a different effect on the dividing cell were used. This system had the advantage not only of making a 'two pronged' attack on the tumour itself but also of reducing the overall toxicity of a cytotoxic schedule since advantage could be taken of the differences in toxicity that exist between the different groups of drugs.

A further advance was made when intermittent chemotherapeutic regimes were introduced. They were based on the work of Howard Skinner of the USA, in 1964, who studied the effects of chemotherapy on mice injected with L1210 leukaemia cells. He showed:

(a) that the percentage of a leukaemic cell population killed by a given dose of a drug was virtually constant and *not* a fixed number of cells;

(b) that the proportion of cells killed is proportional to the dose, assuming a sensitive malignant cell population; and

(c) that the rate of replication of tumour cells appears to be fixed, so that after the death of a proportion of them, unlike normal tissue cells, the growth rate of the remainder does not accelerate to make up for the deficiency.

This latter finding is of great importance since it indicates that the continuous use of a cytotoxic agent does not make optimum use of its potential since the reduction of tumour mass, if the drug is given in tumouricidal doses, will eventually be accompanied by signs of toxicity which may necessitate the cessation of treatment. In theory, by intermittent therapy it should be possible to eradicate the tumour without causing too much damage to the body as a whole. However, the timing of intermittent therapy is critically important; too short an interval between courses may result in evidence of systemic toxicity whereas too long an interval may allow the tumour to recover completely.

Intermittent therapy, now generally used in tumour therapy, apart from reducing the overall toxicity of a chemotherapeutic programme allows higher individual doses of the appropriate agents to be given, thus increasing the proportion of cells killed with each course of treatment. However, despite the theoretical advantages of this type of therapy the vast majority of tumours cannot be completely cured because—

1   The response of a tumour depends upon the growth fraction. Whereas in Skinner's experimental model the growth fraction was nearly 60 per cent in solid tumours, it may be as low as 10 per cent, and since chemotherapeutic agents can act only against dividing cells, the bulk of cells in the average solid tumour, excluding the lymphomas, are resistant.

The small growth fraction in solid tumours is partially explained by the degree of hypoxia within the centre of the tumour which leads to a diminished growth rate and also to poor penetration of the tumour by the agents used.

2   The effects of chemotherapy also depend upon the cell loss factor. A tumour with a large growth fraction and a high cell loss factor is much more vulnerable than a tumour with low growth fraction and small cell loss factor.

Since a clinically detectable tumour is a 'late' tumour, few can be cured. There is, however, a growing body of opinion in favour of treating a patient from whom the primary tumour has been eliminated by surgery by adjuvant therapy in an attempt to control occult metastases.

The protagonists of adjuvant therapy point out that the optimum time to produce tumour kill is at the point at which the tumour cell population is small, a period usually associated with the highest growth fraction. The arguments against adjuvant therapy are—

1   the difficulty of selection;
2   the fact that many patients may be treated unnecessarily;
3   that the long-term adverse effects of such treatment may be undesirable.

1.4   GENERAL PHENOMENA ASSOCIATED WITH NEOPLASIA

General manifestations exist in a wide variety of malignant conditions. They may be classified as follows—

1   **Dermatological markers**

(a)   *Pigmented macules*

Circumoral pigmented mucosal and skin lesions due to an increase in the number of melanocytes in the basal layers of the epidermia and melanophores in the upper dermis are an external marker of the Peutz-Jegher syndrome.

This condition is inherited as a Mendelian dominant characteristic and, in addition to the macules, there is diffuse polyposis of the small bowel. The view has been expressed that these lesions of the small bowel are congenital defects and are hamartomas rather than true neoplasms. The evidence for this view is based on the normal histological arrangement of the cells in the mucosa of the polyps and the fact that such polyps do not become malignant, in marked contrast to the polyps associated with polyposis coli.

(b)   *Neurofibromatosis (von Recklinghausen's disease)*

In this disease, irregular, often large, brown pigmented patches, the so-called café-au-lait spots, appear on the skin. The condition is familial and is inherited as an autosomal dominant, although sporadic cases do appear. In addition to the pigmentation, tumours of nerves develop. These are composed of a proliferation of nerve sheath cells, mainly of Schwann cell origin. In some tumours it may be very difficult to identify axons, making it impossible to distinguish them from fibromata. The nerves involved are those to the skin; in some patients bilateral acoustic nerve neuromata develop and, in addition, abnormalities of bone growth, meningiomata and phaeochromocytoma are found. Neurofibroma in this condition may eventually become sarcomatous.

2   Disturbance of the skin and skeletal muscle

(a)   *Dermatomyositis*

This disorder affects the skin, muscles, and blood vessels, the cutaneous lesion resembling that of a non-specific inflammation such as lupus erythematosus or scleroderma. In the muscles there is a coagulative necrosis, and a predominantly round cell infiltration is found around the smaller arteries. The symptoms of dermatomyositis are usually muscular weakness associated with tenderness and, in some patients, Raynaud's phenomenon. Arthralgias are common at the onset and may recur. Laboratory examination shows changes appropriate to muscle damage. Approximately 30 per cent of all patients suffering from dermatomyositis between the ages of 50 and 70 years have disseminated malignant disease, usually arising from the gastrointestinal tract and, less frequently, the bladder or bronchus. If the tumour can be completely eradicated the condition passes into remission.

(b)   *Epidermal cysts*

Multiple epidermal cysts, associated with multiple osteoma and the development of desmoid tumours following surgery, are the external marker of Gardner's syndrome.

This condition is inherited as an autosomal dominant and is composed of the above tumours together with multiple polyps in the colon. Unlike the polyps of the small bowel these have a strong tendency to become malignant, usually early in adult life.

(c)   *Palmar-plantar keratoderma*

This is a thickening of the skin of the palms and soles, particularly over areas subjected to pressure, occasionally seen in association with carcinoma of the oesophagus.

(d)   *Corn-like keratoses*

More profuse on the extremities, these keratoses may be produced by exposure to carcinogenic agents such as trivalent arsenic. Induration, inflammation, or ulceration indicate that they have progressed to squamous cell carcinoma.

(e)   *Bowen's disease*

This condition is an intraepidermal cancer *in situ* which in both macroscopic and microscopic appearance resembles Paget's disease of the nipple. Approximately 25 per cent of patients with this condition develop primary systemic cancer within five years unless the cause is a local irritant such as arsenic.

(f)   *Acanthosis nigrans*

This is a form of hyperkeratosis which produces a velvety thickening of the skin of the neck, groins, and axillae. The thickened areas are usually pigmented and become grey or black with a mamillated surface on which warty excrescences develop. The condition is associated with malignant tumours of the gastrointestinal tract or lung.

(g)   *Generalised pruritis*

This is rare but its occurrence in the absence of severe obstructive jaundice suggests the presence of a reticulosis.

3   Effects of malignancy on the central nervous system

(a)   *Carcinomatous neuromyopathy*

This condition leads to proximal muscle-wasting together with weakness and loss of the tendon reflexes. The extremities of the limbs are often spared and, as a result, a patient may be unable to lift his legs from the bed and yet dorsiflexion of the foot remains powerful. Some patients suffering from this condition are very sensitive to muscle relaxants. Neuromyopathy is often associated with severe cachexia but there is no relationship. Severe cachexia can be associated with minimal changes and the converse may equally be true.

Less common types of neuromyopathy are—

   (i) Polyneuritic variety.
  (ii) Cerebellar.
 (iii) Sensory.
 (iv) The myasthenic syndrome (Eaton Lambert), in which repeated stimulation of the muscle produces a decreasing number of action potentials.

Neuromyopathy is relatively more common in patients suffering from carcinoma of the bronchus, ovary, and breast, approximately 15 per cent of men with lung cancer, and 16 per cent of women with ovarian cancer developing this syndrome.

(b)   *Multifocal leukoencephalopathy*

This condition is associated with widespread cerebral disease of the cortex which may be severe enough to produce hemiparesis, quadriparesis. aphasia, ataxia, dysarthria, or dementia. It is found particularly in association with lymphoma and leukaemia.

(c)   *Myasthenia gravis*

This may have its basis in malignant disease, particularly when it is associated with a myopathy.

4   Endocrine disturbances

Specific tumours may produce specific hormonal syndromes, e.g.

(a)   *Gastrin-secreting tumours of the islet cells of the pancreas, the gastrinoma*

Intractable duodenal and jejunal ulceration may result from the excessive gastrin production of tumours arising from the delta cells of the pancreas. This syndrome was first described by Zollinger and Ellison in 1955 and the underlying nature of the condition was confirmed more recently as the assay of gastrin levels in the blood became a feasible proposition.

(*b*)   *Insulin-secreting tumours of the islet cells of the pancreas, the insulinoma*

These tumours arise from the beta cells of the islets and result in the development of episodic hypoglycaemia; this diagnosis should be suspected when attacks of faintness or even unconsciousness bear a constant relationship to food intake.

(*c*)   *Serotonin-producing tumours of the small intestine, carcinoid tumour*

Serotonin, 5-hydroxytryptamine, is produced by the argentaffin cells of the small bowel. Excessive secretion of this hormone by a carcinoid tumour causes a variety of symptoms including intermittent flushing and episodic attacks of diarrhoea. The diagnosis is normally confirmed by measuring the excretion of the degradation product, 5-hydroxy-in-dole-acetic acid, in the urine.

(*d*)   *Catechol amine-producing tumours of the adrenals, the phaeo-chromocytoma*

These tumours produce a variety of symptoms depending on the relative proportions of adrenaline and nor-adrenaline that are secreted. Commonly, intermittent attacks of hypertension occur at first, but as the condition becomes more severe a sustained hypertension develops.

(*e*)   *Growth-hormone-producing tumours of the anterior hypophysis, the eosinophil adenoma*

Excessive production of growth hormone after epiphyseal fusion has occurred by an eosinophil adenoma produces acromegaly, characterised by the striking physical changes most noticeable in the face, skin and skeleton and especially in the skull, hands and feet.

(*f*)   *Cortisone or aldosterone-producing tumours of the adrenal cortex*

The former produces Cushing's syndrome characterised by increasing proximal obesity, hypertension, and hirsutism, the last-named causing Conn's syndrome, in which muscle weakness, polyuria, headache and polydipsia are the commonest symptoms.

19

(g) Perverted hormonal behaviour

Some tumours that normally would not be expected to produce hormonal effects may indeed do so. Characteristic of this group is the oat-cell tumour of the bronchus which may produce corticotrophin. This, in turn, stimulates a continuous excessive secretion of cortisol leading to a marked elevation of the plasma 11-hydroxycorticoids, far higher than that seen in the classic Cushing's syndrome. This results in a hypokalaemic alkalosis together with muscular weakness, carbohydrate intolerance, thirst and polyuria. Hypertension and oedema may follow due to sodium retention. The classic features of Cushing's syndrome do not usually have time to make their appearance in patients suffering from bronchial carcinomas because their life expectancy is so short.

Other tumours, however, may be associated with Cushing's syndrome, among which are thymoma and medullary carcinoma of the thyroid. Spontaneous hypoglycaemia is sometimes observed in patients suffering from mesothelioma and liver cancer. The reason is unknown but one hypothesis that has been put forward is that these tumours consume abnormal quantities of glucose because of their high metabolic activity. Another curious occurrence is the occasional excessive production of TSH by hydatidiform moles and chorion carcinoma, leading to hyperthyroidism.

5   Pulmonary osteoarthropathy

This condition of marked clubbing of the fingers, together with pain and swelling of the wrists and ankles, is seen in association with bronchial cancer and pleural mesothelioma. The former tumour may be small, peripheral and operable, resection relieving the syndrome.

6   Thrombotic complications

(a)   The classic thrombotic episode associated with neoplasia is that first described by Trousseau in 1865, of recurrent superficial and deep venous thromboses which undergo spontaneous remission. Trousseau's sign is seen most commonly in patients suffering from tumours of the pancreas, lung, or stomach. The syndrome is called thrombophlebitis migrans.

(b)   Rarely, a non-bacterial thrombotic endocarditis is found in widespread malignant disease. It is caused by platelet aggregations on valves that have undergone necrosis. The common associated tumour is a mucous-secreting adenocarcinoma.

(c)   Very rarely, widespread malignant disease is associated with disseminated intravascular coagulation. This produces afibrinogenaemia together with spontaneous bruising and bleeding, a tendency made worse by the consumption of platelets at the areas of coagulation.

7   Raynaud's phenomenon

The production of cryoglobulins in some patients suffering from multiple myelomatosis, lymphoma and, occasionally, metastatic cancer may lead to the development of Raynaud's phenomena.

8   Generalised cachexia

Although this is one of the common manifestations of widespread and terminal malignancy, the precise cause may be difficult to identify. In gastrointestinal tumours, loss of appetite, bleeding, and sepsis may all play a part, together with some mechanical hindrance to eating. Some tumours such as carcinoid and medullary thyroid cancers are associated with increased intestinal motility and, hence, malabsorption. The latter could also be caused by gastrointestinal cancers that infiltrate the lymphatic and venous systems. Nevertheless, in the vast majority of patients there is no clear explanation of this phenomenon.

9   Fever

Certain tumours such as nephroblastoma, carcinoma of the renal tubules (von Grawitz) tumour and the lymphomas are, in the total absence of any infection, specifically associated with pyrexia. Indeed, in patients with a pyrexia, the cause of which still remains unknown after prolonged investigation, attention should be given to the possibility of an underlying tumour.

10   Metabolic abnormalities

(a)   Hypercalcaemia

Hypercalcaemia may occur in association with any tumour that results in bone resorption or destruction. Thus, it is found in hyperparathyroidism, in association with metastatic bone disease, and, very rarely, in the production of parathyroid hormone-like substances by tumours.

Metastatic tumours able to establish themselves in bone must be capable of causing the dissolution of bone. Experimental work has shown that such tumours can cause the release of calcium from living bone even when this is placed some distance from it, an effect blocked by aspirin, possibly because this drug blocks prostaglandin synthetase.

The symptoms of hypercalcaemia in metastatic bone disease may vary between mild or severe. Mild malaise, aching bones and constipation, followed as the condition progresses by mental depression, psychoses, coma, and death.

21

(b)   Disturbances of purine metabolism

The rapid turnover of cells in some tumours increases the release of the breakdown products of purine and pyrimidines. The resulting rise in the blood uric acid causes the development of gout and uric acid stones in the renal tract. This is a disturbance most commonly seen in the leukaemias rather than the surgical tumours.

1.5   BLOOD TRANSFUSION HAZARDS

The hazards associated with blood transfusion are fortunately rare. Some which previously were commonplace, such as thrombophlebitis and sepsis at the site of administration, have almost disappeared because rubber donor tubes have been replaced by disposable plastics. Other hazards such as incompatability have become less frequent as refined methods of grouping and cross-matching have been introduced.

Specific hazards

1   *Air embolus*

An air embolus can be introduced only if blood is being transfused into the patient under pressure which is usually achieved by pumping air into a glass donor bottle by means of a Higginson's syringe connected to the inlet. If this system is in use it must be kept under close observation to ensure that the fluid in the transfusion bottle never falls below the level of the exit tube to the recipient's vein.

An air embolus produces a frothy air lock in the right ventricle and pulmonary artery, and as a result, the blood pressure falls, the pulse becomes rapid and thready, and a millwheel murmur can be heard over the pericardium.

Management. Once this complication is recognised the tube leading from the bottle must be clipped to prevent further ingress of air and the patient turned on to the left side. The introduction of plastic donor sets has eliminated this hazard.

2   *Overtransfusion*

Cause. The circulation can easily be overloaded by too great a volume of transfused blood in the neonate with a relatively small blood volume, or in a patient suffering from cardiopulmonary disease. When a patient is grossly anaemic and surgical intervention is imperative, blood with a packed cell volume of 65 to 75 per cent should be used within 24 hours of the removal of the excess plasma.

Overtransfusion results in heart failure and the development of pulmonary oedema and, later, peripheral oedema.

Prevention. This complication can be avoided by continuous monitoring of the central venous pressure. When pulmonary oedema inadvertently occurs during or soon after a transfusion, it should be treated by diuretics and amminophylline and, if necessary, venesection.

3   *Febrile response*

A febrile response to blood transfusion is still relatively common although the use of disposable plastic materials has reduced both incidence and severity.

The causes of febrile reaction include—

(*a*)   infusion of pyrogens, usually from a rubber administration set;
(*b*)   transfusion of incompatible blood;
(*c*)   after multiple transfusions, the development of antibodies to platelet, white cell or plasma protein fractions;
(*d*)   use of infected blood.

Prevention. Most febrile reactions have been eliminated by the use of plastic disposable storage bags and donor sets. When multiple transfusions are necessary, red cells alone may be transfused, freed of all other factors by repeated washing.

4   *Incompatible transfusion*

Cause. An incompatible blood transfusion occurs when—

(*a*)   donor cells are administered to a recipient whose plasma contains isoantibodies capable of damaging them. This is the typical 'mismatched' transfusion that may be due to technical error or poor labelling of donor blood or recipient;
(*b*)   donor blood itself contains sufficient antibodies to haemolyse recipient cells;
(*c*)   red cells of reduced viability, usually due to poor storage conditions, are administered.

Any of these situations leads to haemolysis which may be intravascular if brought about by antibodies that are haemolytic *in vitro*, or extravascular when produced by antibodies that cannot haemolyse *in vitro*.

23

Intravascular haemolysis leads to an increase in the circulating haemo-globin, which is bound by the plasma protein, haptoglobin, until the amount exceeds 100 mg/100 ml, after which the excess circulates in the blood stream and is excreted in the urine. Haem separated from the haemoglobin molecule combines with albumin to form methaemalbumin.

Clinical syndrome

1   *Symptoms*

An incompatible blood transfusion usually gives rise to symptoms within 20 minutes. A feeling of warmth may spread up the limb into which the transfusion is being administered, followed by rigors, flushing and fever. Tightness develops in the chest and severe hypotension may occur. The cause of the constricting pain in the chest is unknown but two explana-tions have been advanced: first, that agglutinates block the pulmonary blood vessels; second, that histamine-like substances constrict the pulmonary vessels and bronchioles.

2   *Renal effects*

The effect of a mismatched transfusion on the kidney depends upon its condition before the transfusion. Organic renal disease or gross physio-logical disturbance produced by severe dehydration, hypovolaemia, hypotension or anoxaemia results in haemoglobin or its degradation products producing a severe renal lesion.

Although haemoglobin itself may block the tubules, a major factor causing renal damage appears to be the stroma of the damaged red cells. There is an antigen antibody reaction in the kidney which produces renal ischaemia, later followed by renal failure.

3   *Intravascular coagulation*

Disseminated intravascular coagulation may occur. The severity appears to be proportional to the degree of haemoglobinaemia.

Treatment. Immediate action when confronted by a suspected reaction is to stop the transfusion and remove a sample of blood from the patient and from the transfusion.

The recipient blood should be centrifuged and the supernatant plasma examined for haemoglobin and bilirubin. An attempt should be made to enforce an osmotic diuresis by the administering 100 ml of 20 per cent mannitol, and if the blood volume is still deficient transfusion should be continued with dextran.

If the physiological disturbance becomes an organic lesion and there is renal failure the steps described in *Tutorials in Surgery*, section 1.2 must be instituted.

Viral hepatitis

The hepatitis virus conveyed by blood transfusion has an incubation period of between 50 to 150 days as compared with 15 to 50 days for the incubation of infectious hepatitis.

Following incubation, jaundice of varying severity and duration develops and, occasionally, death from liver failure ensues or the patient develops posthepatitic cirrhosis.

The specific marker for serum hepatitis is the Australia antigen. If blood containing the Australia antigen is transfused, clinical hepatitis is possible. The concentration of antigen reaches a peak soon after the beginning of the disease. It seems probable that all Australia antigen positive subjects are carriers of the virus although in only about one-third has the virus been detected.

Characteristically, the antigen disappears during convalescence but between 1 and 2 per cent of the healthy indigenous population carry the antigen for longer periods. For this reason all blood is now tested for the antigen and, if found positive, is discarded.

The Australia antigen has gained a sinister reputation in dialysis units, but its significance is probably related to the diminished resistance to infection of patients requiring dialysis, and the exposure of staff to large quantities of blood. Nevertheless, stringent precautions to prevent contamination with blood from patients requiring dialysis should be taken.

Transmission of other diseases

(a) Malaria

The malarial parasite is able to survive for days or weeks in blood stored at 4°C. Therefore, the only positive way to prevent transmission is to avoid using as a blood donor any person who has lived in an endemic area, or to screen such donors carefully.

(b) Syphilis

Spirochaetes cannot survive at blood bank temperatures of between 2° to 6°C for longer than three to four days. This alone has reduced the incidence of transfusion syphilis. In addition, blood is routinely tested by one or other of the serological techniques although this is not necessarily a complete safeguard because some 35 per cent of individuals suffering from primary syphilis are serologically negative.

Citrate and potassium intoxication

540 ml of stored blood contains 120 ml acid – citrate – dextrose and as a result, when massive transfusions are necessary, citrate intoxication may occur.

Dangerous levels can be reached during exchange transfusions in the newborn or when more than 5 litres of blood are administered to an adult. The results are a hypocalcaemia, a fall in pH and a prolonged QT interval. The non-specific cardiac depression of citrate intoxication can be avoided by giving 10 ml of 10 per cent calcium gluconate for every 1 litre of transfused blood. The effects of citrate intoxication are made considerably worse by the presence of impaired liver function. This has led to the suggestion that such patients should be given packed cells, rather than whole citrated blood.

In fact, citrate intoxication is usually combined with high plasma potassium concentrations but potassium poisoning alone may occur after large transfusions of stored blood because normal red cells contain 100 mEq/litre (100 mmol/litre) of potassium and during prolonged storage this gradually leaks from the cells, so that at the end of 14 days the plasma concentration of potassium may have reached 200 mEq/litre (200 mmol/litre).

Immunisation

If an Rh negative patient is transfused with Rh positive blood there is an even chance that anti-D antibodies will develop. In the male, the only danger is that further transfusion may lead to a haemolytic reaction. In the female this hazard is also present but, in addition, if she becomes pregnant and the fetus is Rh-positive, the child may be affected by haemolytic disease of the newborn.

1.6 VARIOUS TYPES OF SKIN GRAFT

Classification

1 *Biological.* Skin grafts may be classified according to their origin. An *isograft* or *autograft* is composed of skin moved from one part of the body to another on the same individual. A *homograft* or *allograft* is a graft transferred from one individual to another, and, lastly, a *heterograft* is a graft transferred from one species to another.

In the human, a homograft can survive indefinitely only in certain biological conditions, e.g. when the graft is between identical twins or a genetic chimera. In the latter, a crossed placental circulation *in utero* leads to both twins having a mixed cell population. Thirdly, homografts will survive in patients suffering from agammaglobulinaemia. The duration of survival and the speed of rejection of either skin or visceral allografts varies in different species. In the rabbit, allografts of skin are abruptly rejected on or about the fifth day, the change in skin coloration and texture that marks the rejection taking place in a matter of hours. In the human, the reaction is slower to develop and less intense, and a skin graft obtained from a closely related human, e.g. if the transfer is from a mother to her baby, the rejection of the graft may be delayed for as long as three hundred days without special treatment. The survival of visceral grafts may be prolonged by the use of immunosuppressive agents but these are never used in connection with skin grafts.

2 *Anatomical.* Skin grafts may be free or attached. A free skin graft is one in which the skin is detached from one site and transferred to another, whereas a flap or pedicle graft is a portion of skin and subcutaneous tissue raised from underlying tissues and separated, except for a predetermined area through which the blood supply is channelled.

With the development of microvascular surgery new graft techniques have become available. Applied to skin, grafts can be taken from areas such as the groin, forehead or digit and transferred to the hand, head and neck, lower limb and thorax. These so-called microvascular free flaps are transferred from the donor site and the vascular supply of the graft is directly anastomosed to the arteries and veins of the recipient area.

FREE SKIN GRAFTS

Other than the microvascular free flap referred to above, free skin grafts are normally classified according to their thickness.

1 Thin or thin razor grafts, once known as Thiersch grafts

These grafts are the thickness of tissue paper and are cut just deep to the stratum germinativum by means of a Watson or Braithwaite knife or a dermatome. The outstanding advantage of this graft is the high percentage area of 'take' that can be expected.

The graft laid on the donor area is cemented into position by the plasma that exudes under the graft, coagulates, and forms fibrin. Endothelial loops then invade the graft, and by the fourth or fifth day fibroblasts replace the layer of leucocytes in the interface between graft and recipient area. The vital time, during which the life of this graft is in danger, is between two and five days.

Two disadvantages are inherent in this type of graft—

(*a*) It is *exceedingly* vulnerable and readily destroyed if the recipient area is infected with either *Streptococcus pyogenes* or *Pseudomonas aeruginosa.*

(*b*) The graft contracts in the months that follow healing.

27

The use, therefore, of this type of graft is in the main limited to that of a biological dressing agent such as is required after extensive burning or skin loss due to trauma.

2 Intermediate or split thickness grafts

These grafts are intermediate in thickness between the thin razor and full-thickness grafts (see below). They may be cut by the means previously described, and will 'take' on a granulating wound, on freshly denuded bleeding bone, and on periosteum. One disadvantage of thicker grafts of this nature is the tendency for hyperpigmentation to develop. However, as the graft becomes thicker the tendency for scarring and contracture in the recipient area diminishes while increasing in the donor area. The donor areas chosen for such grafts are the non-hairy portions of the inner arm, the thigh, and abdomen.

Technique of cutting split thickness grafts

When a Watson or Braithwaite knife is used the skin of the selected donor site is first lubricated and then flattened and stretched taut between two flat boards. The operator normally holds one board in his left hand just in advance of the knife edge. As the skin is removed, punctate bleeding ensues, but if fat lobules appear in the donor site the pressure on the cutting edge must be relaxed or the angulation of the blade adjusted.

After split thickness grafts have been taken the donor area may be re-used, at least once, usually within three weeks, the interval before the second cut being determined by the thickness of the skin removed. Epithelialisation of the donor site takes place from the ubiquitous adnexal structures that traverse the skin perpendicular to its cutaneous surface. Split thickness grafts can also be stored for periods of up to four weeks in a temperature of 4°C.

3 Full thickness grafts

These are composed of the total thickness of the skin.

(a) Free grafts

Small full-thickness grafts succeed only if all the subcutaneous tissues have been removed from the deep surface. They are useful when the recipient area must not contract or when the colour of the transplant is important. Favoured donor areas are the postauricular skin, the supraclavicular fossa, and the inguinal crease lateral to the pubic hair.

Such grafts must be carefully removed by dissection, carefully shaped, and carefully sutured into position, the donor area usually being covered by a thin razor graft.

(b)   Pinch grafts

These are often known as Reverdin grafts, after the originator, but they are now only of historical interest. They were cut by lifting a small circle of skin with a needle point and cutting off the resulting protrusion. The result was a small disc of skin of full thickness in the centre and tissue paper thin at the periphery. This type of graft produced both ugly recipient and donor areas and has, therefore, been abandoned.

(c)   Flap transfer or pedicle flaps

These are used wherever it is useful to have a fat pad beneath the skin, the main indications for their use therefore being—

  (i) in circumstances in which there have been large areas of skin loss and full thickness replacement is necessary, e.g. on the leg or face;
 (ii) to cover avascular structures and protect them from infection, e.g. an open joint, exposed bone or tendon;
(iii) as a prelude to orthopaedic reconstruction.

A single pedicle flap has one peripheral attachment and may be transplanted by advancement, rotation or interposition.

Forward advancement (Fig. 1.1). The simplest form of skin advancement is that used in an area in which the soft tissues are loose and abundant, the long axis of the wound corresponds to the lines of minimal tension, and the edges of the wound may be approximated without tension, sutures maintaining this position during healing. However, if an elliptical wound is situated in an area of the body in which the surrounding tissues are under tension, then approximation is facilitated by undermining the skin edges of the wound through the subcutaneous tissues, thus releasing the superficial tissue from its deep attachments. By this procedure two advancement flaps become established.

For larger defects a more elaborate method must be used although the principle remains the same, i.e. a flap attached only at one end is advanced to fill a defect. The inherent elasticity of the skin permits a certain amount of advancement, but under no circumstances should the flap that is formed by outlining three sides by means of incisions be stretched like a rubber band. Several methods of facilitating advancement have been devised, the two most commonly used are—

(a)   the excision of triangles of skin at the base, a method first described in 1838 (see Fig. 1.2A)

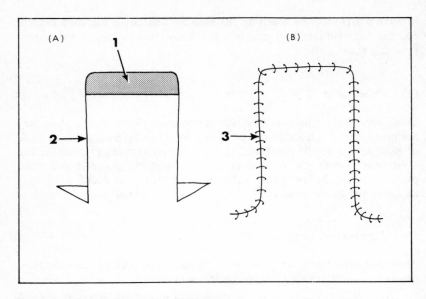

Fig 1.1 Skin graft – forward advancement
1. Skin defect 2. Line of incision 3. Finished effect

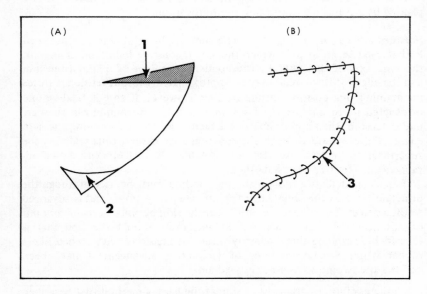

Fig 1.2 Skin graft – rotation flap
1. Skin defect 2. Triangle excised 3. Finished effect

(*b*)   alternatively the flap may be elongated by a Z-plasty technique at the base.

Rotation flap (Fig. 1.2). This is frequently used to advance skin from the neck to the cheek. A rotation flap will normally stretch into a wound if the flap is so cut that the curvilinear perimeter is at least four times greater than the distance to be advanced. Advancement is facilitated by a back cut which is really the excision of the Burow triangle.

Interpolation flap. By this technique tissues near to but not adjacent to the wound are interposed into it. An example is the use of a temporal flap to restore the lower eyelid.

The survival of single pedicle flaps depends on meticulous control of the blood supply to the flap. At all times the blood supply should be adequate, and in order to ensure this the length of the pedicle should not exceed the base; if there should be any fall in blood pressure there may be a disastrous thrombosis of the blood supply. If a longer flap is required the blood supply can be improved by delaying the flap. This is done by partially raising the flap from its bed and then replacing it *in situ,* a man-oeuvre that ensures the flap obtains its blood supply from the pedicle, and one particularly useful when dealing with lower limb flaps in which a delay of 10 to 21 days is always an advantage. Too long a delay, however, must be avoided because the graft slowly begins to pick up a blood supply from its periphery.

Once the flap has been positioned it cannot obtain an adequate blood supply from the recipient area for at least two weeks, hence the pedicle of the flap must be left undisturbed for this length of time.

4   **Tube pedicle grafts** (Fig. 1.3)

This type of graft is frequently raised from the abdomen, the inner aspect of the arm, the acromiopectoral region, or the anterior aspect of the thigh.

In general, the length of the tube should not be greater than twice its width at the time of its actual formation. Furthermore, the long axis of the tube must be parallel to the direction of the cutaneous and sub-cutaneous vasculature. The advantages of a tube pedicle graft are its resistance to infection and the final cosmetic appearance of the recipient area.

The most important feature of a tubed pedicle graft is that it is the ideal method of delaying before transfer. Normally, movement of the tube should be carried out three or more weeks after its formation. Such a tube may be moved over considerable distances; for example, a tube raised on the abdomen can first be attached to the wrist and then brought down to the lower limb or upwards to the face. Because most people are right-handed the left wrist is normally used. The complications of a tube pedicle graft are usually those associated with bleeding. If a haematoma

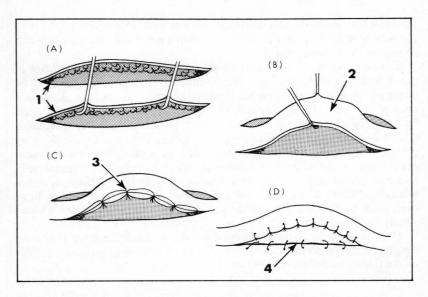

Fig 1.3   Limits of pedicle graft construction (Gillies) 18 cm long if at least 5 cm in width
1. Parallel incisions   2. Flap raised   3. Tube completed   4. Skin defect closed

develops in a tube it must be removed otherwise it may severely interfere with the blood supply and could, at worst, produce loss of skin.

5 Microvascular free flap

This type of graft involves removal of a full-thickness graft together with its arterial supply and draining vein. So long as these are between 1 to 3 mm in diameter, by using an operating microscope it is possible to perform adequate end-to-end vascular anastomoses.

With groin flaps the superficial circumflex iliac artery is used. Around the eye, the anterior superficial temporal artery together with the supra-orbital vein and anterior temporal vein are available. The cause of failure of this type of flap is also vascular and it is usually due to thrombosis of the arterial supply. It is particularly likely to happen if there is a discrepancy between the thickness of the subcutaneous tissues of the donor skin and the recipient site, which produces kinking of the artery. Alternatively, there may be venous thrombosis. Early intervention and re-anastomosis is required because this type of flap does not withstand secondary ischaemia. This type of graft surgery has recently been used for the replacement of digits that have been cleanly severed from the hand; and occasionally it is possible to reimplant a whole limb.

1.7 PAIN AND ITS RELIEF IN THE SURGICAL PATIENT

THE ANATOMY OF PAIN PATHWAYS

1 Specific receptors

These are structures designed to lower the threshold of excitability for one type of stimulus and raise it for all others. They are divisible into—

(a) free nerve endings occurring either in skin, muscles, joints or viscera.
(b) encapsulated organs, such as the Meisner's corpuscle subserving touch, the Krause end bulb subserving cold, and, in muscle, the muscle spindle that subserves proprioception.

2 Nerve fibres

The nerve fibres carrying the sensation of pain are found in the γ fibres of A fibres, the B fibres, and the C fibres.

The cell bodies of the sensory part of the spinal nerves are in the dorsal root ganglia; peripheral fibres arising from peripheral receptors pass as somatic sensory fibres in the appropriate spinal nerves, while fibres from the viscera travel via the sympathetic nerves to the sympathetic chain and enter the spinal nerves via the white rami communicantes. Although travelling in the sympathetic nerves they are not a part of the autonomic system.

3 Within the spinal column

The proximal fibres from the ganglia form the posterior nerve roots which enter the spinal cord as the medial and lateral bundles. The former consist of large myelinated fibres which pass via the dorsal columns to the basal spinal nucleus, whereas the lateral bundle contains a majority of C type fibres which enter the dorsal horn of grey substance and form the dorso-lateral tract of Lissauer. Fibres from Lissauer's tract pass to the substantia gelatinosa in which they terminate and synapse with the internucial neurones. From these second order neurones fibres pass back into Lissauer's tract and synapse many times with other neurones, fibres running up and down for many segments.

The second order neurones cross the ventral white commisure to the opposite side of the cord to form the anterolateral spinothalamic tract, decussation occurring within a few segments of their entry into the cord. The spinothalamic tract then ascends unbroken through the brain stem to the posteriolateral ventral nucleus of the thalamus, gathering fibres as it ascends until eventually a laminated structure is formed. This lamination is especially marked in the cervical region although the actual arrangement is extremely variable.

4 Central connections

Having reached the thalamus, pain-carrying fibres radiate in a diffuse fashion to—

(*a*) the paracentral cortex which is associated with precise localisation;
(*b*) the frontal lobes, particularly to the orbital surface, these pathways being involved in the emotional content and response to the experience;
(*c*) to the temporal lobes which are concerned with the identification of pain and memory patterns.

Multiple connections with the reticular activating system also exist, and with rostroreticular neurones which regulate the amount of cortical stimulation and influence the localisation and memory for pain.

5 Chemical central control of pain perception

Recently, polypeptides known as the enkephalins and endorphins have been identified in the periaqueductal system, the substantia gelatinosa and the thalamus, hypothalamus and midbrain. These compounds are blocked by the narcotic antagonist nalaxone and both are released in the experimental animal by direct stimulation of the periqueductal grey matter or nerve stimulation. Their release can be inhibited by narcotics, and their catabolism may be blocked by the administration of tricycyclic drugs.

Despite the relatively sound knowledge regarding pain pathways there is, as yet, no one theory to account for all the complexities of pain perception.

Pain due to surgical conditions may be of somatic or visceral origin. The latter is often short-lived and may be relieved according to its aetiology in a variety of ways—

(a)   by intermittent use of an appropriate analgesic, e.g. renal or biliary colic;

(b)   by medical treatment of the cause, e.g. the use of antacids in the treatment of heartburn due to reflux and hyperacidity;

(c)   by excision of the affected viscus, e.g. acute appendicitis.

Whatever the cause of the pain, psychological factors play a large part in its intensity.

In any person, the threshold for pain perception, which is that intensity of stimulus at which pain is perceived, is fairly constant but the upper threshold or tolerance to pain can be considerably altered by psychological factors. Thus, anxiety can lead to a greater experience of pain while the hysteric exaggerates his or her experience. An introverted patient generally has a low threshold and reduced tolerance but makes few complaints, while the extrovert who has a high threshold and increased tolerance displays a high level of complaint.

All these factors must be taken into account when dealing with the problem of pain.

ANALGESIC RELIEF

Analgesic agents are commonly divided into those of mild or intermediate potency and the narcotic group, the last-named being subdivided again into naturally occurring and synthetic products. The disadvantage of narcotics is their addictive nature and their somatic and psychologically adverse effects. However, none of these, other than constipation, is of great importance if the patient has reached the terminal stages of disease, and at this point doses several times the accepted norm should be given without hesitation if it makes the patient's remaining life more tolerable.

The three minor analgesics in common use are aspirin, paracetamol, and dextropropoxyphene hydrochloride. Because of the psychological aspects of pain perception already referred to, psychotrophic drugs may be used to potentiate these analgesics. These include the minor tranquillisers such as diazepam, the major tranquillisers such as chlorpromazine and promazine, and antidepressants such as phenelzine and amitriptyline hydrochloride. Either group may be used, depending upon which appears the more appropriate at the time.

INTRACTABLE PAIN

Intractable pain may be defined as pain of insufferable intensity and of long duration. Although the commonest reason for intractable pain is visceral malignant disease, several other causes exist—

(a) pain due to bony metastases, which may be relieved by hormone therapy or irradiation;
(b) disease of peripheral nerves, e.g. causalgia;
(c) occlusive vascular disease.

The methods devised to deal with intractable pain include—

1   Neurolytic agents

The use of subarachnoid or intrathecal injections of alcohol for the relief of chronic pain was first reported by Dogliotto in 1930. At present, 10 per cent phenol in glycerine is more popular because it carries slightly less risk, although alcohol is still used for injection into the trigeminal nerve.

Technique

The patient must be positioned with the affected painful side uppermost, lying midway between the lateral and prone positions because alcohol is less dense than cerebrospinal fluid. If, however, phenol in glycerine is used, the patient should lie with the affected side downwards. To relieve bilateral pain the patient should be laid prone with the back arched in order to raise the dorsal roots to a high level, and alcohol should be injected.

The volume of absolute ethyl alcohol administered should be limited to 1 ml and the injection should be given at the spinal level subserving the pain, remembering that the spinal cord segment and the vertebral level progressively separate from above downwards. Following the injection the patient should remain stationary for a period of at least one hour.

Kuzucu reported that the period over which relief was obtained was very variable, usually in the region of three to four months, although it may sometimes last for a year.

When using phenol in glycerine the injection should be made as close as possible to the spinal segments and roots requiring destruction. A contact time in excess of five minutes is necessary, and the exact volume needed varies with the site of the injection; to block the sacral nerve roots, approximately 0.3 ml is required and to block the upper lumbar area 0.6 ml. These doses are usually administered in two separate portions at five-minute intervals.

Following an injection of phenol there is often loss of touch and other cutaneous sensations, including awareness of pin prick. The method appears to be most effective for relieving well-localised pain and least effective in relieving midline or extensive bilateral pain. The degree of success is variable, as low as 25 per cent in some series and as high as 60 per cent in others.

The major complications of this method are muscular weakness, bladder disturbance and hypoaesthesia over the blocked dermatomes.

2   Non-operative techniques for relief of pain

(a)   Barbotage

This is the withdrawal and rapid replacement of cerebrospinal fluid through a wide-bore needle. Relief of pain for up to three months has been reported. The method is dangerous if practised in the high cervical and thoracic regions.

(b)   Intrathecal injections of either ice-cold or normothermic 10 per cent saline

Pain relief of up to two months duration has been reported. The disadvantage of the method is the need for a general anaesthetic because of distressing symptoms produced by the injection.

3   Operative treatment of intractable pain

(a)   Posterior rhizotomy

When used for relieving pain in the thoracic region it is essential to section two roots above and below the affected segment. Thus, five roots must be exposed and a major laminectomy performed. Sensory deprivation of the trunk is relatively unimportant, but denervation of the extremities produces grave difficulty in co-ordination.

The same principle can be applied to trigeminal neuralgia when the appropriate sensory root of the trigeminal nerve is divided after exposure through the middle fossa. If a fractional section is performed by avoiding the first division, corneal anaesthesia and, thus, the possibility of damage to the eye, can be avoided. The motor root is also spared, hence facial weakness does not occur.

(b) Open anterolateral cordotomy

The usual site for this operation is the upper thoracic or cervical region. It is of limited application because intractable pain is often bilateral, and bilateral cordotomy is prone to produce bladder complications. If the operation is performed the section must be made on the side opposite to the pain, and because the pain and temperature fibres cross the cord over 5 or 6 segments the sensory level affected is 5 or 6 segments below the level of section.

The advantages of cervical cordotomy are technical. At this level the cord does not fill the vertebral canal and it is easier to rotate it by exerting traction on the dentate ligament. A knife is then used to cut the lateral spinothalamic tract which lies immediately anterior to it. However, a high cervical cordotomy may damage the descending respiratory pathways which lie close to these tracts. Pain relief usually follows section of the spinothalamic tract for approximately six months.

(c) Percutaneous cervical cordotomy

This operation was described by Mullan. It is applicable to pain within the distribution of cervical 5 to sacral 5. The technique does not require general anaesthesia but the patient must be very co-operative. The principles of the operation are as follows—

A needle is inserted just below and behind the mastoid process, and its position in the subarachnoid space relative to the dentate ligament is radiographically determined. Once it is thought that the correct position has been reached a trial stimulation is performed, the distribution of the subjective sensation indicating the probable distribution of pain relief following coagulative destruction.

(d) Intracranial procedures

Leucotomy, although capable of diminishing the affective element of pain, does not remove its perception; further, personality changes associated with this operation may be severe. Leucotomy for the relief of intractable pain has, therefore, been replaced by operations on the limbic system such as cingulotomy.

(e)   *Sympathetic denervation in the treatment of causalgia*

Causalgia is an intense intractable pain in the hand or foot of a limb in which the peripheral nerves have been injured. It often begins immediately after injury, but tends, in many patients, to improve slowly with the passage of time.

It is described by the sufferer as a superficial burning pain associated with a persistent deeper aching pain. The pain is usually aggravated by physical or emotional stimuli and the affected limb is often protected from all injury.

In many patients there are associated trophic and vascular changes in the affected part, indicative of autonomic disturbance. The skin is glossy, skin temperature is higher than normal, and the soft tissues may be atrophic. The cause of causalgia is unknown but one recent explanation is that ephasses, electrical synapses, are formed between different types of nerve fibre that have come into contact with one another because of peripheral nerve injury; against this theory is the fact that demyelination of nerve fibres does not immediately follow injury.

The treatment of causalgia is sympathectomy, but before operation it must be established that there will be a favourable response by performing a procaine block of the appropriate ganglia. In the upper limb, the second thoracic ganglion should be infiltrated, and for the lower limb the second, third and fourth lumbar ganglia. In general, the most favourable response is said to follow early interference before the pain pattern is imprinted on the central nervous system.

Following sympathectomy the original disability due to the nerve lesion persists and, in some patients, after a variable period of time, even after an apparently satisfactory result, the causalgia returns, often after a lapse of a year.

In addition to these more orthodox methods of pain relief perceptual manipulation can be achieved by hypnosis, transcendental meditation, or the use of hallucinogenic drugs or, alternatively, the central nervous system can be stimulated by a variety of means such as percussion, used for a painful amputation stump or transcutaneous nerve stimulation by intermittent passage of an electric current.

2 General Surgery

2.1   THYROIDITIS, DIAGNOSIS AND TREATMENT

HASHIMOTO'S THYROIDITIS (LYMPHADENOID GOITRE)

This condition was first described by Hashimoto in 1912, but it was not until the late fifties that Doniach and Roitt, later supported by Burnett, produced the first hypothesis on the aetiology of the condition.

Clinical presentation

Typically, the patient suffering from Hashimoto's disease is a middle-aged woman who presents with either a diffuse, smooth, rubbery-hard goitre or, alternatively, an asymmetrical enlargement of the same consistency. In the early stages of the disease signs of mild hyperthyroidism may be present but in the later stages hypothyroidism develops. In some patients, discrete enlargement of the associated cervical lymph nodes may occur.

Interestingly, an atrophic variant of the disease, which is associated with a small goitre, becomes increasingly frequent with age. This atrophic type is five times commoner in females than in males whereas the goitrous type is nearly twelve times commoner in the female and has a peak incidence in the sixth decade.

Hashimoto's disease may co-exist with pernicious anaemia and even in the absence of overt anaemia circulating antibodies against gastric parietal cells may be found.

Pathology

Macroscopic

The gland is discrete, showing an exaggeration of the normal lobular pattern. The cut surface, usually whitish in colour, appears extremely avascular compared to a normal gland.

Microscopic

The chief changes are—

1 dense intrafollicular infiltration of the gland by plasma cells and lymphocytes in which, in some patients, germinal centres may appear;
2 oxyphilic changes in the cytoplasm of the follicular cells, together with follicular destruction;
3 increasing amounts of fibrous tissue within the gland:
4 there appears to be some association between Hashimoto's disease and non Hodgkin's lymphoma.

Aetiology

The concept initially suggested by Doniach and Roitt was based on an immunological premise. They suggested that the components of the thyroid were hidden from immunologically competent cells in the crucial period during which immunological tolerance was developing; that is, the period during which the body learns to distinguish between self and non-self. Any damage to the thyroid, therefore, might release materials that could be antigenic. Regarded as foreign to the individual's normal immunological system, they would provoke an antibody response which, in reacting against thyroid tissue, would set up a chain reaction in the gland, producing continuing damage.

The arguments that have been marshalled against this concept include—

(a) Studies on the basement membrane surrounding the thyroid follicles. These show that the membrane of the follicle is much more tenuous at 24 weeks in utero than in Hashimoto's disease, a finding which suggests that the immunological system of the developing fetus is, of necessity, familiar with the various constituents of the normal thyroid follicle.

(b) Studies on the level of thyroglobulin and related materials in the newborn. These have shown that thyroglobulin or a closely related chemical substance is actually circulating in the blood of the newborn infant.

(c) Thyroglobulin excretion in the adult. In the adult, the hormones T3 and T4 are split off from thyroglobulin by hydrolysis emerging from the outer poles of the follicle cells into the thyroid capillaries. However, a number of studies have shown that a small amount of thyroglobulin escapes hydrolysis and is taken up by the lymph surrounding the thyroid acini. This finding alone suggests that the immunological system is continuously exposed to thyroglobulin throughout life.

(d) Studies on thyrotoxic patients treated with radioactive iodine. ^{131}I in large doses produces extensive damage to the thyroid cells and yet, following treatment, the serological status of the patients does not change.

(e) Some patients suffering from thyrotoxicosis have demonstrable antibodies in their blood, others do not. Treatment does not convert serologically negative patients into positive nor does it elevate the titre of antibodies in those serologically positive before treatment.

As a result of this evidence the term autoimmune thyroiditis is now used to define a condition characterised by the presence of circulating thyroid antibodies. There is now no longer any implication that these substances have any causal relationship to the thyroid disorder although in general terms there is a correlation between the titre of antibodies and the degree of lymphoid and plasma cell infiltration of the thyroid tissue.

Although the casual triggering agent remains unknown it is now believed that the circulating T immunocytes (thymus dependent lymphocytes) come in contact with antigen and provoke the formation of IgG antibodies in the serum.

At least four different IgG antibodies reacting with different components of the thyroid cell have been described; of these the thyroid microsomal antibodies are probably the most important, for in tissue culture they are highly cytotoxic to human thyroid cells in the presence of complement. The antigen antibody reaction results in the release of lymphokines which attract lymphocytes of the B type into the area of conflict; the result is a diffuse infiltration of the thyroid with lymphocytes and the formation of lymphoid follicles which produce more B lymphoctyes.

The antigens of the thyroid include thyroglobulin, the cytoplasmic microsomal antigen, the CA2, or second colloid antigen, and a cell surface antigen. The various antigens and antibodies are found in a variety of combinations and permutations. The thyroglobulin antibody will react with all colloid extracts except abnormal forms of thyroglobulin such as those formed in dyshormonogenetic goitres.

Investigations

Since the histroy and clinical examination provide such convincing evidence of the diagnosis, all the laboratory tests described below may be regarded as confirmatory—

1 Erythrocyte sedimentation rate; this may be elevated.
2 Uptake of ^{131}I or ^{132}I; this may be low, normal or raised, depending on the stage of the disease. At an early stage uptake commonly falls to subnormal values. During this period the serum TSH may be increased and the response to exogenous TSH may be subnormal, indicating a diminished thyroid reserve.
3 Plasma TSH, this may be normal or elevated.
4 Serum T4 concentration. Usually normal in the early stages of the disease, it gradually falls to subnormal levels as the thyroid reserve diminishes.
5 Antibody tests. The tests used to detect antibodies are—

(a) tanned red cell or coated latex particle (coated with human thyroglobulin);
(b) haemagglutination tests;
(c) precipitin tests;
(d) occasionally, complement fixation and immunofluorescent techniques may be used.

The antibodies disclosed include antithyroglobulin and microsomal antibodies and anticolloid antigens.

The sensitivity of these various tests is such that less than 1 per cent of patients suffering from this form of thyroiditis escape detection.

Results

Although antibodies are present in high titres in patients suffering from Hashimoto's disease and spontaneous myxoedema they are also present in at least 50 per cent of patients suffering from primary thyrotoxicosis. Indeed, a titre of greater than 1/25 to thyroglobulin is present in 16 per cent of normal women and approximately 2 per cent of normal men. However, the microsomal antibodies are more discriminating, being associated only with immune disease. In patients suffering from primary thyrotoxicosis the presence of antibodies is usually accompanied also by focal lymphocytes within the gland and a greater than normal probability of becoming myxoedematous following treatment.

The presence of antibodies does not necessarily rule out the possibility of malignancy, especially because of the relationship between autoimmune thyroiditis and lymphosarcoma, and if the diagnosis is open to any doubt an open biopsy should be performed.

Treatment

The usual treatment of Hashimoto's disease in the absence of pressure symptoms is the administration of L-thyroxine 0.2 to 0.3 mg/day orally. The treatment is continued throughout life, and in about half the patients the gland regresses. Myxoedema is also avoided, but in any case the gland may remain static for many years.

It should also be noted that approximately 10 per cent of sufferers from Hashimoto's disease develop Addison's pernicious anaemia, and possess antibodies to the gastric parietal cell in their serum. A careful watch should, therefore, be kept at intervals on the peripheral blood count and the serum vitamin B12 level.

SUBACUTE THYROIDITIS

Also known as viral, granulomatous, giant cell or deQuervain's thyroiditis.

Aetiology

This condition is thought to result from a viral infection of the thyroid gland. It often follows an upper respiratory tract illness, in some patients mumps and, in addition, the Cocksackie, ECHO and adenoviruses have been implicated. Support for this hypothesis comes from the occasional demonstration of viral antibodies.

Clinical presentation

The classic feature of this disease is the gradual or sudden appearance of pain in the region of the thyroid accompanied in some cases by a fever. The disease is rare, tends to occur equally in both sexes and affects the young rather than the old. The patient is usually euthyroid but occasionally transient hyperthyroidism occurs, presumably due to the abnormal amounts of T4 liberated from the gland as it undergoes destruction.

On palpation the thyroid is usually slightly to moderately enlarged, firm, and in the early stages, exquisitely tender. Occasionally the overlying skin may be warm and red. The disease usually subsides within a few months leaving no residual deficiency of thyroid function.

Pathology

The histopathological picture is totally different from that of Hashimoto's disease. The condition tends to be patchy in distribution. In affected areas the follicles are infiltrated with cells predominantly of the mononuclear type. These follicles show disruption of their epithelium and partial or complete loss of colloid, together with fragmentation of the basement membrane. In addition, cores of colloid may be seen surrounded by multinucleate giant cells. As the disease resolves so the histology of the gland returns to normal.

Investigations

1 Erythrocyte sedimentation rate, usually elevated.
2 ^{131}I uptake, usually very low in the early stages of the disease.
3 T4 concentration high at first then subnormal.
4 Circulating antibodies, usually present in low titre during the active phase of the disease, disappearing as the disease subsides.

Treatment

This is mainly symptomatic; the transient hyperactivity may be controlled by β-blockers. If pain is a feature, the administration of high doses of prednisone, 20 mg three times a day, may help.

CHRONIC THYROIDITIS

Also known as woody thyroid or Riedel's stroma, chronic thyroiditis is a rare disease.

Some textbooks state that the condition is the end stage of Hashimoto's disease but clinical experience does not confirm this since the disease apparently begins in a hitherto healthy gland and may, within a few weeks, convert the thyroid into a rock hard mass the borders of which cannot be distinguished from surrounding structures.

Pathology

Macroscopic examination at operation confirms that the gland is avascular greyish in colour with apparent extension of the pathological process into surrounding tissues.

Microscopy confirms that the gland is affected by a diffuse fibrosis which resembles that observed in retroperitoneal and mediastinal fibrosis.

Investigation

In nearly every case a surgical open biopsy is required to exclude the presence of anaplastic thyroid cancer. Thyroid function tests are relatively valueless since function remains normal and there are no thyroid antibodies.

Treatment

Occasionally, a limited isthmic resection is required to relieve tracheal compression. The author has found that high doses of steroids tend to bring the condition under control and to reduce the neck stiffness which is a constant source of complaint. However, the condition is so infrequent that this remains a clinical impression of dubious value.

2.2 THE PATHOGENESIS, MANAGEMENT AND INDICATIONS FOR SURGERY IN CHRONIC DUODENAL ULCERATION

Definition. A chronic ulcer of the duodenum, 99 per cent of which ulcers occur within one centimetre of the pylorus. Commonly solitary, involving either the anterior or posterior wall, in 15 per cent of cases two ulcers are present, usually on the opposing walls of the duodenum, producing the so-called 'kissing' ulcers. In approximately 16 per cent of patients suffering from duodenal ulceration a concomitant gastric ulcer is also present.

Incidence

The true incidence of duodenal ulceration is difficult to establish. In industralised societies the incidence is greater in males than in females and tends to increase with advancing age so that the percentage of the population affected by the disease, either active or inactive, may rise to 10 per cent in males and 5 per cent in females over the age of 50.

Pathogenesis

The development of duodenal ulceration is dependent upon the interaction of many factors—

(*a*)   provoking ulceration is the digestive action of pepsin and acid;
(*b*)   preventing ulceration are the mucosal defensive factors.

While much is known about the former, the latter still remain to be quantified.

Acid factor

In the majority of patients suffering from duodenal ulceration, gastric hyperacidity can be demonstrated both in the basal, unstimulated state, the BAO, and following stimulation by such high doses of histamine, or its synthetic analogue pentagastrin, that the maximum possible acid output is attained (MAO). There is, however, a considerable overlap between apparently normal individuals and those suffering from duodenal ulceration. Furthermore, the degree of hypersecretion does not necessarily correlate with the duration or severity of the symptoms or with the frequency of complications.

Not only do patients suffering from duodenal ulceration tend to secrete more acid in response to chemical stimuli but they also over-respond to all other known types of stimuli, especially food and the hypoglycaemia provoked by insulin. Three hypotheses have been advanced to account for the hypersecretion observed in the majority of patients suffering from duodenal ulceration—

1 an increase in secretogenic stimuli acting on the stomach, i.e. an increased vagal or hormonal drive on the acid producing parietal cell mass;
2 an increase in the total quantity of secretory units within the mucosa which secrete greater than normal quantities of acid even in the absence of any specific stimulus;
3 a decrease in the sensitivity of the antral or duodenal mechanisms that normally act to inhibit excessive acid output.

The first hypothesis is supported by the abolition of acid hypersecretion by vagotomy, provided that antral stimulation is avoided and that the resulting gastric juice contains large quantities of pepsin.

There is, however, considerable evidence that the quantity of acid it is possible to secrete is directly related to the size of the parietal cell mass, a view first put forward in 1960 by Card and Marks. The relationship, however, is not so simple as it at first appeared. Following their initial findings, these investigators went on to establish that the parietal cell acid output varied according to the underlying type of ulceration. Thus, the 'maximum acid output' per billion parietal cells in patients suffering from duodenal ulceration was 28 mmol/hr and for gastric ulceration only 18 mEq/hr. However, a direct relationship is present between the basal secretion and maximal acid output, a correlation suggesting that the differences in acid secretion between patients may be regulated in part by vagal drive.

In absolute terms the size of the parietal cell mass in a normal male (Cox, 1952) is 1.18×10^9 which results in an output of 11.6 mmol of acid/30 min under maximally stimulated conditions. In a patient suffering from a duodenal ulcer, however, the number of parietal cells rises to 1.9×10^9 cells and the maximal secretory response to 22.9 mmol/30 min.

Why this increase in parietal cell mass should occur remains doubtful; the suggestion has been made that it is due to work hypertrophy due to persistent stimulation. The rate of gastric emptying is also a factor of possible significance since it is greater in patients suffering from duodenal ulceration than in normal individuals. Rapid gastric emptying decreases the buffering action of a meal and thus allows chyme with a lower pH than normal to enter the duodenum.

However, although acid together with pepsin undoubtedly play a major role in the development of ulceration this cannot be the only factor because relapses and remissions are found in the same patient, even though the BAO and MAO remain unchanged. Thus, it is not yet clear whether gastric hypersecretion, when present, is the cause of duodenal ulceration or whether it is merely one rather easily detected facet of the pathophysiological disturbances underlying ulceration. In conditions such as the Zollinger Ellison syndrome there can be little doubt as to the importance of the 'acid equation' since in this condition, characterised by continual gastric hypersecretion, duodenal and even intestinal ulceration always develop.

Mucosal resistance

The second factor that must be considered is the resistance of the mucosa to the action of acid and pepsin. Abnormalities in the mucosal protective mechanisms, in the form of a defective layer of mucus over the surface of the mucosa, have been sought in ulcer patients for a long time. It is considered by many that the high incidence of blood group O with non-secretor status in patients suffering from duodenal ulceration indirectly reflects some abnormality of the mucus. However, the relevance of the blood group secretor status and the different composition of the gastric mucus to the pathophysiology of duodenal ulceration has not been established. No significant advances have yet been made concerning the relationship between mucus and 'protection' of the duodenal mucosa against acid and pepsin. There is also little information concerning the mucosa of the duodenum itself, the mucosal abnormalities described in patients with established ulceration providing little information regarding the pre-ulcerative state of the mucosa.

Vascular hypothesis

The fact that the majority of peptic ulcers occur singly and are situated either on the anterior or posterior walls of the first part of the duodenum strongly suggests that some localising factor is at work. It has been recently suggested that such localisation occurs because of the poverty of the vascular supply to the first two centimetres of the duodenum, which is supplied, at least in part, by end arteries of extramural origin. In support of this theory it is of interest that the vascular pattern of the duodenum of the dog, a species that does not normally suffer from duodenal ulceration, is entirely different from the human.

Symptomatology

The symptoms associated with uncomplicated duodenal ulceration are pain and vomiting. Characteristically, the severity of the pain is extremely variable, depending partially on the psychological make-up of the patient and the severity of the disease. It is normally provoked by hunger and, therefore, will often wake the patient in the early hours of the morning, and it is aggravated by alcohol, smoking, and dietary indiscretion. The attacks are often self limiting and intermittent regardless of treatment, lasting for days, weeks, or months and then improving, apparently spontaneously. An interesting study was made in 1964, by Fry, who entered general practice after a surgical career. He studied the incidence and course of duodenal ulceration in a large general practice and found that once a symptomatic ulcer developed, increasing disability often followed for 5 to 10 years after which inexplicable remission occurred.

Vomiting is frequent during severe attacks and is usually caused by pylorospasm rather than organic stenosis. Characteristically, it will often lead to immediate symptomatic relief, presumably because the acid stimulus to the bare nerve fibres in the ulcer crater is removed by emptying the stomach.

Effect of medical therapy

Early investigations into the effect of any form of therapy on the healing of duodenal ulcers was bedevilled by the periodic nature of the symptoms that commonly occur in the absence of treatment and by the absence of any precise diagnostic method that would allow a true appreciation of the state of the duodenal mucosa. The latter has now been overcome by the perfection of the fibreoptic duodenoscope which allows, with little danger to the patient, repeated visualisation of the first part of the duodenum.

1   *Diet*

Although it is frequently stated that a patient suffering from duodenal ulceration should be placed on a bland diet, meals being eaten in small quantities and at frequent intervals, there is little experimental evidence to support this advice. Nevertheless, when a patient is actually suffering from symptoms he often appreciates such a diet although there is no evidence that to continue with it once he is asymptomatic is in anyway helpful. Tobacco smoking should be stopped, if possible, since there is a considerable body of evidence supporting the contention that cessation of smoking accelerates the healing of gastric ulcers and it has, therefore, to be assumed that the healing of a duodenal ulcer may be accelerated in a similar fashion.

2 Antacid therapy

The traditional treatment of duodenal ulceration is by antacids. However, although there is little doubt that the symptoms can be temporarily relieved by administration of such drugs, included among which are, magnesium carbonate and trisilicate, aluminium hydroxide gel, calcium carbonate, and bismuth subnitrate, there is no evidence that they actually accelerate the rate of healing. In order to achieve this it would be reasonable to assume that they would have to be administered in such high doses that the gastric acid was completely neutralised. This, for practical purposes, is almost impossible to maintain in a male seeking to continue working. Thus, in order to neutralise 50 mmol of gastric juice hourly it has been calculated that it would be necessary to administer between 4 to 5 g of calcium carbonate, magnesium oxide, or sodium bicarbonate hourly.

Complications of antacid therapy. Such high doses of calcium cause hypercalcaemia in approximately one-third of patients and when the total dose of magnesium oxide exceeds 4 g/day severe diarrhoea always occurs. Sodium bicarbonate, because of its solubility, immediately relieves pain but the relief is of short duration and is followed by a rebound phenomenon resulting in a temporary increase in the volume of acid secreted.

Other complications following prolonged and excessive antacid medication include the milk-alkali syndrome in which renal insufficiency gradually develops, together with renal calcification and alkalosis. Excessive calcium carbonate ingestion may eventually lead to hypercalcaemia because calcium chloride can be absorbed and this will be followed by hypercalciuria and the formation of calcium containing stones.

Non-absorbable antacids containing magnesium and aluminium hydroxide may impair the absorption of phosphorus which, in turn, leads to an increased resorption of skeletal phosphorus and calcium, producing the clinical syndrome of anorexia, weakness, bone pain and malaise.

3 Anticholinergic drugs

The administration of anticholinergic drugs is the pharmacological equivalent to surgical vagotomy. The effective drugs in this group include dicyclomine hydrochloride, hyoscyamine, propantheline and poldine hydrochloride, all of which competitively inhibit vagal stimulation, thereby reducing gastric secretion and motility. The majority have an atropine-like effect and, therefore, when taken in excess will produce dryness of the mouth, dilatation of the pupils, slowness of micturition and occasional vomiting. However, a single dose of 2 to 3 mg of a drug such as poldine hydrochloride will reduce gastric secretion within one to two hours of its administration for several hours. A further advantage of the atropine-like drugs is that they are also antispasmodics and, therefore, tend to relieve the pylorospasm which is considered by many to make a significant contribution to the pain of duodenal ulceration. Such drugs should be used with caution in patients suffering from prostatic hypertrophy, coronary insufficiency, and glaucoma and because of the significant lack of evidence that these drugs as a group are particularly effective in promoting ulcer healing; they are now seldom used.

4   Antidepressant drugs

The drug, trimipramine, a tricyclic antidepressant has been shown to lower the secretion of both gastric acid and pepsin, possibly due to an antihistaminic effect. Trials using endoscopic control have shown that a daily dose of 50 mg of this drug significantly increases the rate of healing of chronic duodenal ulcers as well as diminishing the symptoms. The common adverse effects are drowsiness and dryness of the mouth.

5   Prostaglandin E, analogues

These drugs remain of theoretical rather than practical interest although it has been demonstrated in a double blind prospective study that such compounds significantly increase the rate of healing of duodenal ulcers when compared with a placebo. This is presumably because they produce an effective but, unfortunately, short-lasting suppression of acid output by direct action on the parietal cell mass. However, in the trial referred to above a significant number of patients developed such severe diarrhoea that the dose of the drug had to be reduced.

6   Histamine H2 receptor antagonists

Histamine is a drug with many sites of action, and when the first class of antihistamines were developed about 30 years ago they were found to be capable of blocking some of the effects of histamine such as allergic reactions, and also, of pharmacological properties largely independent of their antihistaminic activity, including anticholinergic, antiadrenaline and antiserotonin effects. However, this first group of drugs, which included promethazine and cyproheptadine hydrochloride, had no effect on gastric secretion and it was therefore assumed that there were two classes of histamine receptor, H1 and H2. The H2 receptor antagonists were finally discovered by Black in 1972, and three drugs have now been described, burimamide, metiamide and cimetidine, of which the last appears to be the least toxic and the most effective in the clinical field. Metiamide was abandoned when it was discovered that in some patients bone marrow depression, albeit reversible, was induced. This effect was thought to be due to the presence of a thiourea residue in the metiamide molecule, and in cimetidine this has been replaced by a cyanoguanidine group which appears to render the drug less toxic but more potent than its predecessor.

It has now been shown that a dose of 300 mg of cimetidine will inhibit the basal acid secretion, in patients suffering from duodenal ulceration, by as much as 95 per cent for a period of at least five hours, and when administered prior to retiring to bed it appears to reduce acid secretion by at least 80 per cent throughout most of the night. The effect is, however, mainly on the volume of secretion. In a patient eating normally and taking four doses daily, gastric pH nevertheless remains below 2 for much of the time, but the acid secretion is sufficiently reduced to allow ulcer healing. It is believed that cimetidine acts by direct inhibition of histamine on acid secretion and by inhibiting the potentiating action of histamine on that acid secretion stimulated by gastrin and acetycholine.

Clinically, in a succession of prospective randomized double blind trials it has been shown that cimetidine is clearly superior to a placebo, an ulcer healing rate of 71 per cent being achieved in a total number of 348 patients as compared to only 37 per cent in a placebo treated group. Although symptomatic relief does not correlate exceptionally well with the healing rates in all the trials that have been reported, symptomatic relief was significantly higher than in the placebo group. The recommended dose of this drug appears to be 200 mg thrice daily plus 400 mg at night, and on such a regime there is an 80 per cent chance of the ulcer disappearing in four weeks.

No haematological abnormalities have been seen but the question of hepatotoxicity remains in some doubt. A few men have noted breast soreness and enlargement after several months treatment but without any evidence of hormonal or other sexual change.

However, although cimetidine has been shown to be effective in producing symptomatic remission and ulcer healing it does not impart any long-term benefit in that the cessation of treatment is followed, in the majority of patients, by relapse since the underlying causes of the ulcer remain unaltered. However, it has been shown that if cimetidine therapy is continued, particularly if the drug is taken immediately prior to retiring to bed, there is a significantly lower relapse rate than in placebo treated patients up to one year. However, once again, even after controlling acid secretion for this relatively long period relapse occurs once therapy is discontinued.

7   *Miscellaneous non-surgical treatments*

(*a*) Gastric irradiation.
(*b*) Gastric freezing.

Both these methods have received considerable attention in the past, both have been shown to be capable of reducing the secretion of acid and pepsin, but both methods have been abandoned for a variety of reasons, the chief of which are the inherent dangers and, secondly, the relapse rate, which is high because of the ability of the gastric mucosa to regenerate even after severe damage has been inflicted upon it.

Indications for surgery

1   *Intractability*

This may be defined as an inability to bring about a sufficient relief of symptoms by medical means to render life tolerable for the affected individual. The degree of relief necessary obviously varies considerably in the different socioeconomic groups and in different occupations. Intractability may be due to the action of exogenous factors, e.g. an unhappy marriage or lack of job satisfaction. On the other hand, it may be due to the severity of ulceration; a posterior duodenal ulcer penetrating the pancreas will often produce severe and intolerable back-pain as well as profound dyspepsia.

Occasionally, intractability is due to the presence of multiple endocrine adenomatosis (MEA) of the type in which pituitary, parathyroid, and islet cell tumours occur. The presence of intractable ulceration, one facet of the Zollinger Ellison syndrome, is evidence that this condition may be present.

2   *Perforation*

The optimum treatment of perforated duodenal ulcers is still in some doubt. Many years ago Herman Taylor suggested that patients who perforate after only a short history of dyspepsia should be treated conservatively, i.e. by gastric suction and intravenous fluids, whereas in the presence of chronic symptoms radical surgery should be performed even in the presence of a perforation, and simple suture should be abandoned. The arguments put forward in favour of such a programme are as follows—

(*a*) in the majority of patients suffering from perforation the ulcer is already 'sealed' by the time of operation.

(*b*) a short history suggests acute ulceration, hence the result of simple suture is not only to implant foreign materials within the wall of the duodenum, thereby exciting a foreign body reaction, but in addition to produce a degree of devascularisation, thereby encouraging the development of chronic ulceration.

In the majority of patients treated by conservative means the progress of the patient can easily be established by clinical examination. If such a conservative regime is used there should be a rapid improvement in the abdominal physical signs within a matter of hours so that a patient admitted complaining of generalised abdominal pain and with generalised rigidity in the evening should be virtually pain free by the following day and the area of rigidity should be confined, if present at all, to the epigastrium.

The opponents of this type of management maintain that it may be followed by the development of a right supra- or infra-hepatic abscess, the former being especially difficult to treat. There is little doubt that this is so, but there is no large-scale series treated conservatively, other than Herman Taylor's original series, which, in fact, states the extent of this problem in numerical terms.

3   *Suture*

The failure of simple suture for the treatment of chronic duodenal ulcers has recently been described in a retrospective study by Playforth and McMahon (1978) who showed that the mortality of this simple operation was of the order of 5 per cent and that 48 per cent of the patients continued to complain of ulcer dyspepsia following recovery, 33 per cent requiring elective surgery.

4   *Pyloric stenosis*

Cictricial contraction of the first part of the duodenum is an absolute indication for surgical treatment. Such a complication is usually accompanied by the development of pseudo-diverticuli which are most pronounced when two ulcers are present. In such saccular pouches all layers of the duodenal wall are represented and occasionally the radiologist screening the patient may mistake such a pouch for a large active ulcer.

In the past, the treatment of choice was regarded as posterior no-loop gastrojejunostomy but it was eventually recognised that this simple procedure, although associated with a low mortality, was, in fact, accompanied by a high incidence of anastomotic ulceration, the ulcer occurring in the proximal part of the efferent loop. It is, therefore, now the practice to perform whatever elective procedure the surgeon would normally use except in the extremely debilitated individual in whom a simple, quick procedure is necessary.

5   *Haemorrhage*

See *Tutorials in Surgery: 1* p.194.

2.3   THE HISTORICAL DEVELOPMENT OF DUODENAL ULCER SURGERY

Gastric surgery for the relief of peptic ulceration arose from the use of operations that were initially performed to overcome obstructive lesions at the pyloric end of the stomach. The original operation of gastro-enterostomy is credited to Wolfler in 1881, but shortly afterwards Rydyier of Poland and Doyen of France described its application for the treatment of cicatricial pyloric stenosis due to duodenal ulceration.

Gastroenterostomy

In its original form, gastroenterostomy was performed by anastomosing a jejunal loop to the anterior wall of the stomach, and it was not appreciated, at first, that the length of the afferent loop was critical to the proper mechanical working of the operation, too long a loop leading to the syndrome of vicious circle vomiting. The posterior 'no-loop' procedure now in common use was developed by Czerny and was immediately adopted by Mayo and Moynihan.

Until the First World War, gastroenterostomy was regarded as the operation of choice for duodenal ulceration, and in the first decade of the twentieth century individual surgeons were reporting personal series of several hundreds of cases.

Those surgeons who practised gastroenterostomy firmly believed that the anastomosis accomplished three things. First, it diverted food from the ulcer, thus avoiding irritation of the ulcerated surface and allowing it to heal. Secondly, it allowed the influx of bile and alkaline pancreatic juice into the stomach, thus neutralising the acid contents. Thirdly, it diverted acid from the pylorus, thus abolishing the jet-stream effect on the first part of the duodenum. It was not, of course, appreciated at the time that several effects of gastroenterostomy mitigated against a good result. These include: the damaging effect of bile on the gastric mucosa by destroying the mucosal barrier; the place of continuous antral alkalinity as a stimulus to continuous parietal cell secretion; and lastly, the fact that the stomach drains through the anastomosis only when the pylorus is completely obstructed.

Nevertheless, many surgeons, including Moynihan, reported exception-ally good results. In 1923 Moynihan published his experiences of ten years of ulcer surgery and recorded his results in 531 cases. He reported a low operative mortality and a satisfactory result in over 90 per cent of patients. In his personal series he reported that the incidence of anastomotic ulcera-tion was only a little over 1 per cent. At that time, of course, jejunal ulcers were considered to be caused by faulty operative techniques such as the use of non-absorbable sutures, rather than unsolved physiological problems.

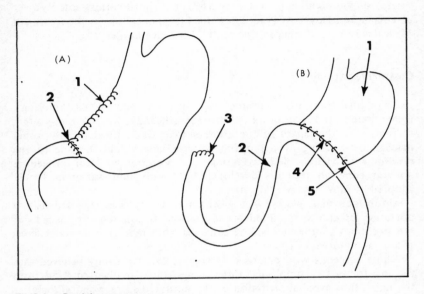

Fig 2.1   Partial gastrectomy
(A)   Bilroth I operation described in 1881
1. Reconstructed lesser curve   2. Gastro-duodenal junction, angle of sorrow, due to possibility of leakage
(B)   Bilroth II described in 1885
1. Gastric remnant   2. Danger point, too long an afferent loop   3. Danger point, rupture of duodenal stump   4. Gastro-jejunal anastomosis   5. Site of recurrent ulceration

Despite this and many similar reports, it was finally appreciated that gastroenterostomy carried a very high morbidity in the way of jejunal ulceration. Many large series showed that recurrent ulceration, usually situated on the efferent loop, occurred in as many as 50 per cent of patients, the incidence being greatest in males under 50 years of age and within the first five years following surgery.

It is also interesting that dumping, which is one of the commoner physiological side effects of gastric surgery, seems to have gone entirely unrecognised by the earlier surgeons, for the first review of this subject did not appear in the literature until 1920. Today, gastroenterostomy is never used alone for the treatment of duodenal ulceration despite its low mortality, even in patients suffering from severe pyloric stenosis in whom it was once regarded as the treatment of choice.

Partial gastrectomy

In 1881, Bilroth successfully removed the pyloric end of the stomach and restored the continuity of the gastrointestinal tract by a direct gastro-duodenal anastomosis (Fig. 2.1A). In 1885, he performed a pylorectomy and then closed the duodenum and restored the continuity of the bowel by anastomosing the jejunum to the stomach remnant (Fig. 2.1B). Following the original description of these surgical techniques, many useless but original anatomical modifications were described. By the end of the First World War both operations were being performed for the treatment of duodenal ulceration and, indeed, the Bilroth II, or Polya gastrectomy, as it came to be known, was the operation of choice from the mid-nineteen thirties to the early sixties.

It was soon appreciated that anastomotic ulceration could not be prevented unless the antrum was resected, and gradually the extent of the gastric resection increased as it became recognised that the smaller the resection the higher the incidence of this complication. However, it was also recognised that too radical a resection eventually culminated in the appearance of the gastric cripple, due to the small stomach remnant, its rapid emptying, and intestinal hurry.

Several decades passed before it was fully appreciated that the Bilroth I type of resection was not as satisfactory as the Polya for the treatment of duodenal ulceration. The main disadvantage of the former was the high incidence of recurrent ulcers astride the anastomosis, despite apparently adequate resection of the stomach; an incidence as high as 28.6 per cent has been reported from some centres as compared to an incidence of 1 to 2 per cent following an adequate Polya resection in which two-thirds to three-quarters of the stomach are removed.

Complications

Both the Bilroth and Polya type of resections are followed by a variety of symptoms and syndromes apart from anastomotic ulceration. These include—

1 Postcibal syndromes, early and late dumping, small stomach syndrome.
2 Bile vomiting.
3 Iron deficiency anaemia, especially in the premenopausal woman.
4 Weight loss probably due to postcibal symptoms.
5 Megaloblastic anaemia.
6 Severe malnutrition following very radical resection.
7 An increased incidence of pulmonary tuberculosis.
8 Cancer of the stomach remnant.
9 Mortality varying between 1 to 5 per cent.

Results

Despite this formidable list of undesirable side effects, approximately 80 per cent of patients subjected to a Polya type of gastrectomy are highly satisfied with the result. Of the remainder, three-quarters regard their condition as improved, and the rest are dissatisfied.

The degree of dissatisfaction in the majority is closely related to the extent of the gastric resection. Visick, a protagonist of radical resection, found that although extensive resection reduced anastomotic ulceration to negligible proportions it was, at the same time, accompanied by a distressing high incidence of postcibal symptoms.

Some of the symptoms and syndromes listed above tend to improve with the passage of time. Thus, early dumping can be expected to improve and even completely disappear, although complete remission may take many months. Other conditions such as bile vomiting may improve, but if it persists, in the majority of patients it can be corrected by dividing the afferent loop and reanastomosing it to the efferent loop at least 25 cm distal to the gastrojejunal anastomosis. If this operation be considered necessary it should always be accompanied by vagotomy, otherwise in about 25 per cent of patients, anastomotic ulceration occurs.

Yet other conditions such as anaemia may require continuous medication and supervision.

Mortality

The mortality of partial gastrectomy varies between 1 and 5 per cent according to the series examined. The chief complication specifically related to partial gastrectomy, which leads to disaster, depends upon the type of operation performed. Following a gastroduodenal anastomosis (Bilroth I), the major problem is leakage from the junction of the reconstructed lesser curve and duodenum, a point known to the Germans as the 'angle of sorrow'. Following a Bilroth II or Polya procedure the chief hazard is rupture of the duodenal stump, a complication that may occur at any time between the 4th and 21st postoperative days. When it occurs early, this complication leads to general peritonitis, and when it occurs later the common manifestation is the development of a right supra- or infra-hepatic abscess, drainage of which leads to a temporary duodenal fistula.

Vagotomy

Truncal Resection

The unphysiological nature of partial gastrectomy and the relatively high incidence of unsatisfactory results led to attempts to control parietal cell secretion by section of the vagi. The first subdiaphragmatic vagotomy was reputedly performed by Exner in 1911, but the operation was only seriously advanced as an alternative to gastrectomy by Dragstedt in 1943. However, at this time the operation was almost immediately abandoned because of the undesirable effects of gastric stasis and the development of secondary gastric ulcers in some 10 to 15 per cent of patients. It was reintroduced, combined on this occasion with a drainage procedure in 1945, again by Dragstedt.

Complications of Vagotomy

The adverse effects of vagotomy and drainage are numerous, for the latter may produce all the symptoms associated with gastrectomy, while the chief complication of the former is diarrhoea. The cause, treatment, and avoidance of this has become the subject of intense discussion.

True vagotomy diarrhoea is episodic, transient, but may be torrential and, therefore, disabling. Many investigators consider that it arises because viscera other than the stomach are denervated.

Particular attention has been paid to the fact that truncal vagotomy causes gall-bladder dysfunction because it interferes with the nerves supplying this organ. It has been shown that, following truncal vagotomy, the gall-bladder enlarges and almost doubles its fasting volume, that it contracts poorly after a fatty meal, and that there is an increased incidence of gall-stones. In addition, the hypothesis has been put forward that when such a dilated gall-bladder does contract it delivers so large a volume of bile into the gut that the small intestine is unable to absorb the bile-salt content, with the result that some bile salts reach the large bowel and there inhibit the absorption of water, salt, and potassium, to produce the watery motion which is so classical of postvagotomy diarrhoea.

This theory is supported by the fact that in many patients the diarrhoea can be controlled by the drug cholestyramine, which binds the bile salts and, secondly, that the incidence of diarrhoea is sharply reduced by performing a selective vagotomy.

Selective Vagotomy

Essentially this operation, as first described in 1948 by Franksson of Stockholm and Jackson of Ann Arbor, consists of dividing the vagi a little lower down on the stomach itself, below the origin of the hepatic branches of the anterior vagus and the coeliac branch of the posterior vagus, so that although the vagal supply to the entire stomach is interrupted the biliary tract and small gut remain innervated.

This operation received enormous attention, particularly from the late Harold Burge in the United Kingdom. The protagonists claimed that it was effective both in terms of a low incidence of recurrent ulceration and a reduced frequency of diarrhoea. However, because this operation is still associated with a drainage procedure, all the consequences of destruction of the pyloric sphincter and rapid emptying of the stomach may follow, such as dumping. It is also interesting to note that not all surgeons are agreed that this operation successfully reduces the incidence of post-operative diarrhoea.

Highly Selective Vagotomy

In 1957, Griffith attempted to denervate, in the dog, the acid-producing parietal cell mass alone, and in 1967 this work was applied to man by Holle and Hart who combined it with a drainage procedure because they failed to realise that when the vagal innervation of the antrum and pylorus is retained, the emptying mechanism of the stomach is unimpaired and a drainage procedure is unnecessary. It was left to Johnson and Wilkinson of Leeds and, simultaneously, Amdrup and Jenson of Copenhagen to realise the true significance of highly selective parietal cell vagotomy or as some prefer to call the operation, proximal gastric vagotomy.

Essentially, this operation consists of dividing all the branches of the anterior and posterior vagal nerves, commonly known as the anterior and posterior nerves of Latarget, from a point distal to the division of the anterior vagal trunk into its hepatic and gastric branches (Fig. 2.2). This division should start at a point on the side of the oesophagus and continue along the lesser curve of the stomach to a point about 7 cm proximal to the pylorus, at which it can be seen that the anterior nerve is dividing to form a 'crow's foot' arrangement as it splits to innervate the antrum (Fig. 2.3).

When performing this operation care must be taken to ensure that the lowermost 5 to 7 cm of the oesophagus has been completely bared of vagal trunks or nerve fibres running to the stomach and that meticulous

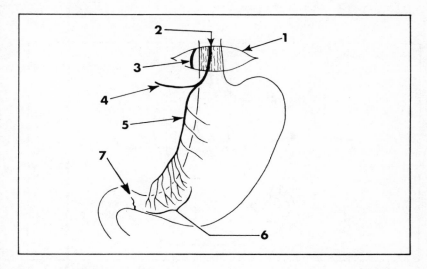

Fig 2.2   Highly selective vagotomy: Start of operation – Exposure of main vagal trunks
1. Transverse peritoneal incision – exposing lower oesophagus and anterior and posterior
vagal trunks   2. Anterior vagal trunk   3. Posterior vagal trunk   4. Hepatic branch
5. Anterior nerve of Latarget   6. Crow's foot   7. Prepyloric vein of Mayo

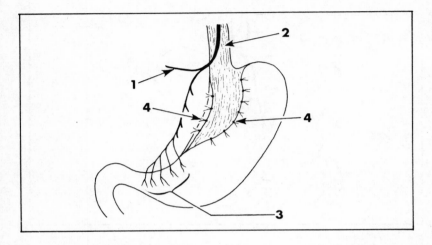

Fig 2.3   Final appearance of operation
1. Hepatic branch of anterior vagus nerve   2. Oesophagus   3. Crow's foot left intact
4. Points of division of branches of anterior and posterior nerves of Latarget

haemostasis is maintained throughout. The advantages of this operation are that by preserving pyloric innervation and, therefore, normal gastric emptying, it should theoretically avoid dumping, and although the antral area retains its innervation it remains in the acid stream and, therefore, cannot release the excessive quantities of gastrin that normally stimulate the parietal cell mass to secrete acid. The basal acid output following this operation is reduced by approximately 80 per cent, and the maximal acid output by about the same degree as it would by truncal or selective denervation.

The protagonists of proximal or highly selective vagotomy maintain that dumping is rare, diarrhoea infrequent, and the incidence of recurrent ulceration no greater than that following partial gastrectomy. The latter claim is, however, open to question. This operation, at the time of writing, would appear to be the operation of choice in the treatment of duodenal ulceration but its general application is somewhat limited by the technical difficulties which are particularly apparent in the obese patient.

Many different series have now been reported in the surgical literature supporting these various contentions. The mortality of the operation is also low, the chief danger being that the severe devascularisation of the lesser cruve, which is necessary to ensure division of all the branches of the anterior and posterior nerves of Latarget, may lead to necrosis of the lesser curve. This complication has, in fact, been reported but, fortunately, its incidence is low.

Miscellaneous methods of treatment

Three other methods, all abandoned, have at various times been used to reduce gastric acidity and so treat duodenal ulceration. The first of these was gastric irradiation, introduced by Bassler, in 1909, who found that a temporary histamine fast achlorhydria lasting for approximately six months could be produced. The temporary nature of the effect of irradiation, which is due to the ability of the gastric mucosa to regenerate, led to a high incidence of recurrent ulceration, 30 to 50 per cent, and this manoeuvre was soon abandoned.

In the late forties, Somervell reported his results using gastric de-vascularisation. This operation was also shown to be followed by large-scale recurrence. Lastly, in 1960, Wangensteen introduced physiological gastrectomy by freezing the stomach with an inflowing coolant at $-17°$ to $-20°C$ for 45 to 60 minutes. However, by 1963, Rufton had shown in a double blind trial that the symptomatic results of sham freezing were precisely the same as those of real freezing, and so this has been abandoned.

2.4   THE PREVENTION AND TREATMENT OF INJURIES TO THE EXTRAHEPATIC BILIARY SYSTEM

Anatomy of the extrahepatic biliary system

A knowledge of the anatomy of the extrahepatic biliary system is essential if damage to it is to be avoided at the time of operation. So many anatomists and surgeons have devoted their time to the anatomy of this region and produced so many differing findings that many of the differences that once were regarded as anomalies can now be taken as mere variations of the normal anatomical arrangement.

In practice, it is probable that these variations and anomalies do not make a very significant contribution to the incidence of ductal injuries and that the more important factor is haemorrhage in the operation field, which appears to the inexperienced operator, to be uncontrollable. This leads him to panic measures, the inexperienced surgeon then, quite incorrectly, attempting to control the bleeding by the use of instruments rather than by packs.

Further, although the anatomy may be perfectly normal the surgeon may misinterpret his operative findings; for example, a normal but narrow common bile duct may easily be mistaken for the cystic duct, particularly if it should separate easily from the other structures contained in the right border of the lesser omentum.

The accepted 'normal' anatomical arrangement of the ductal system

The commonly accepted description of the normal anatomy of this region is as follows (Fig. 2.4):

The right and left hepatic ducts emerge from the liver and join to form the common hepatic duct, in the great majority of individuals in an extrahepatic situation. At a somewhat lower level, the cystic duct enters the common hepatic duct, and below this level the duct, now known as the common bile duct, which is approximately 1 cm in diameter, proceeds inferiorly, posteriorly, and slightly laterally. It passes behind the duodenum and through the head of the pancreas to enter the medial surface of the duodenum at the ampulla of Vater. Recognition of both the common hepatic and common bile ducts is made easier by the presence on their surface of a venous network. The cystic duct is usually easily recognised near its junction with the common hepatic by the presence of the cystic duct lymph node and, in addition, this point also becomes more obvious once tension has been exerted on the gall-bladder by cholecystectomy or sponge forceps. The level of the conjunction may be considered 'neutral' if a reasonable length of the common hepatic and common bile ducts can be identified above and below it.

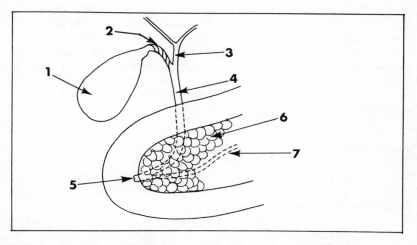

Fig 2.4   Accepted "normal" anatomy of the extra hepatic biliary system
1. Gall bladder   2. Cystic duct with valve of Heister   3. Common hepatic duct
4. Common bile duct   5. Ampulla of Vater   6. Pancreas   7. Duct of Wirsung

Variations in the ductal system

(*a*)   Rarely, the cystic duct joins the right hepatic or the common hepatic at such a high level that an apparent trifurcation is produced (Fig. 2.5A). Either of these anatomical anomalies may cause difficulties at operation, particularly if a stone is impacted at the points of conjunction.

(*b*)   The cystic duct may run parallel with the course of the common hepatic for a considerable distance before joining the common bile duct (Fig. 2.5B), occasionally in the retroduodenal position or even within the pancreas. The cystic may be so tightly bound to the common bile duct that the only indication of the presence of this variation is a shallow groove between the two structures. A second indication that this anomaly exists may be the obvious presence, from the external appearance of the cystic duct, of the spiral valve of Heister which causes, when marked, a series of 'ripples' on the surface of the cystic duct.

True anomalies

1   *The cholecysto-hepatic duct.* Such ducts are rare and are often un-recognised at the time of surgery because they emerge from the gall-bladder bed and immediately join the gall-bladder. During the dissection of the gall-bladder from its bed a duct of this kind can easily be overlooked unless the operator is astute enough to recognise the presence of bile issuing either from the raw surface of the liver or from a small orifice on the hepatic surface of the gall-bladder.

The importance of this rare anomaly is that should it go unrecognised and the duct is left unligatured, in the early postoperative period it may cause an unexpectedly large loss of bile from the wound. Alternatively, it may cause biliary peritonitis or, at a later stage, a subphrenic abscess.

2   *Accessory hepatic ducts.* These are also rare and, if present, usually enter the common hepatic duct proximal to its junction with the cystic duct. As with a cholecysto-hepatic duct, inadvertent damage may lead to postoperative biliary leakage. However, unlike the former, this anomaly should be more easily recognised during the course of dissection.

3   *Fusion of the cystic duct with the right hepatic duct.* Fortunately, this anomaly is also rare, because if it is unrecognised a number of surgical misadventures, including ligation of the right hepatic duct, may await the unwary.

Vascular anatomy

The commonly accepted description of the normal arterial arrangement is as follows (Fig. 2.6):

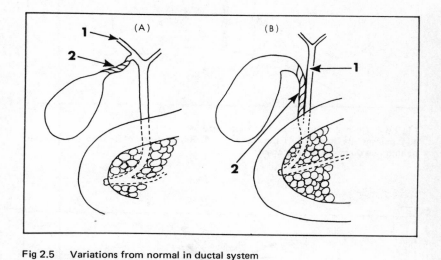

Fig 2.5   Variations from normal in ductal system
(A)   Cystic duct joining the right hepatic duct
1. Right hepatic duct   2. Cystic duct entering right hepatic duct
(B)   Cystic duct running parallel with common hepatic duct for an abnormal distance
1. Common hepatic duct   2. Cystic duct running parallel to and usually adherent to
common hepatic duct over an abnormal distance

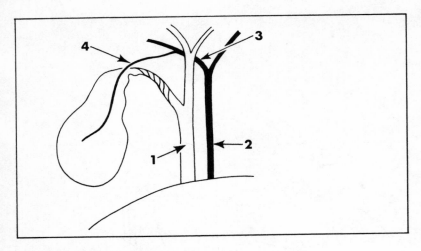

Fig 2.6   Normal arrangement of hepatic arteries
1. Common bile duct   2. Hepatic artery   3. Right branch of hepatic artery passing
behind bile duct   4. Cystic artery

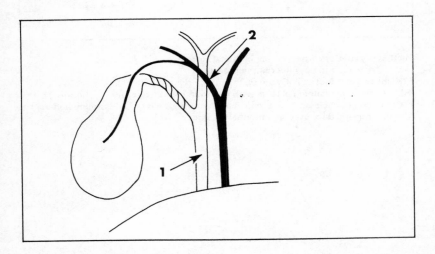

Fig 2.7   Transposition of right hepatic artery
1. Common bile duct   2. Anterior transposition of right hepatic artery

The hepatic artery arises from the coeliac axis artery and passes upwards towards the liver on the medial (left) side of the common bile and hepatic bile ducts. It terminates by dividing into right and left branches which normally enter the hilum of the liver posterior to the right and left hepatic ducts. At some point the right hepatic artery gives off the cystic artery, which passes behind the common hepatic duct before reaching the gall-bladder.

Anomalies of arterial supply

The arterial anomalies are important to the surgeon because, unanticipated and unrecognised vascular anomalies may be the cause of severe bleeding if such a vessel is inadvertently divided before a ligature has been applied. If this should happen, damage to the biliary system could result if attempts to control the haemorrhage are misdirected. Furthermore, although a normal healthy individual is usually unaffected by division and ligation of the right hepatic artery, which is the vessel in greatest danger, in the presence of cirrhosis the result may be fatal.

The common anomalies of the vascular supply to the liver and biliary system in order of frequency are—

1 The presence of an accessory cystic artery. These arteries always arise from the right hepatic artery. Unrecognised, such an artery may be avulsed from the main artery causing severe haemorrhage with all its attendant dangers.

2 Anterior transposition of the right hepatic artery (Fig. 2.7) and hence of the cystic artery. Such an anatomical arrangement should be of little importance, but if the artery crosses the common bile duct at a relatively inferior level it may interfere with its exploration, i.e. cholodochotomy, should this be considered necessary.

3 The 'caterpillar hump' right hepatic artery. This is the least common of the arterial anomalies. The artery, instead of proceeding directly into the hilum forms a loop which bulges laterally beyond the right hepatic duct in either an anterior or posterior position. This anomaly is frequently associated with a short, stubby, cystic artery so that the application of a ligature becomes technically difficult. An alternative source of danger is failure to recognise the anomaly at all, with the result that the vessel is ligated and divided after which the two cut ends may slip from the ligature and cause torrential bleeding.

Causes of injury to the extrahepatic biliary system

The common causes of injury to the extrahepatic biliary system include—

1 Failure to recognise the common duct even in the presence of negligible pathological changes. This can only be defined as 'ham-handed' surgery and should seldom, if ever, occur. Cholecystectomy demands the proper visualisation of all parts of the biliary tract before any ligature or

clamp is applied, or structure divided, and a large part is played in this by the assistants. Remember Moynihan's dictum, it is the assistants who perform the operation. This was, of course, particularly true in his day in which relaxants were unknown. Then, exposure of the biliary tree demanded a full-scale Kocher's incision from the tip of the tenth rib on the right to the costal margin on the opposite side, the incision being placed two fingers' breadth below the costal margin.

2 'Tenting' of the common bile duct at its junction with the cystic duct. This type of injury, in which a cholecystectomy forcep is placed across the right lateral face of the common duct, occurs only if excessive traction is used when attempting to identify and ligate the junction of the cystic with the hepatic ducts. It is also more common when there is little or no pathology of the common duct. An absence of inflammatory change allows it to be more easily displaced laterally by traction from the right free border of the gastro-hepatic omentum.

3 Injury caused by inadvertent clamping during the arrest of unanticipated bleeding. This is now the most common cause of damage to the extrahepatic biliary system and usually follows avulsion or division of the cystic artery or a laceration of the right hepatic artery. Either event is followed by rapid haemorrhage, and the operation field is quickly obscured. At this point the inexperienced operator may well plunge an instrument, such as a Moynihan's cholecystectomy clamp, into the region of the porta hepatitis, damaging either the upper end of the common hepatic duct or one or both hepatic ducts. It cannot be too strongly emphasised that the correct treatment of this type of bleeding is immediate packing of the wound. Patience is then required, waiting, if necessary, up to 30 minutes before slowly removing the pack. An additional manoeuvre, described long ago by the surgeon Seton Pringle, is to compress the hepatic artery in the free border of the hepatoduodenal ligament. The latter has not been found by the author to be of great value.

Less common causes of injury include—

1 Damage during the performance of a partial gastrectomy. This was commoner in the past when this operation, which involves mobilisation of the first part of the duodenum, was in general use for the treatment of severe duodenal ulceration.

2 Operations designed to remove diverticuli from the second part of the duodenum.

How to avoid injury

(*a*)   Obtain an adequate exposure of the area by a generous incision and good retraction.

(*b*)   Define all structures; in particular clearly demonstrate the junction of the cystic duct with the common hepatic duct and the hepatic and common bile ducts proximal and distal to this point.

(c) Should the anatomy of the region be so distorted by disease that (b) above appears impossible, then retrograde cholecystectomy should be performed, removing the gall-bladder from the fundus towards the cystic duct. Unfortunately, this may be far from easy because of bleeding from the liver bed which, however, can be controlled by a second assistant putting pressure on the raw surface with a retractor well-padded with gauze, and advancing the retractor progressively as the dissection proceeds.

(d) In cases presenting overwhelming technical difficulty the inexperienced surgeon should retire from the scene after first performing a cholecystotomy and extracting those stones present in the gall-bladder.

Clinical signs of inadvertent injury

1   *Injuries at the time of operation*

Injuries of the common bile duct made by inadvertent division at the time of operation may be immediately recognised. If so, they should be repaired immediately, splinting the one layer anastomosis of the duct by a T-tube which should be left in situ for about three weeks. Anatomostic breakdown, which would inevitably mean the subsequent development of a stricture, can be demonstrated by means of postoperative cholangiograms performed via the T-tube on the 10th and 16th day.

2   *Injuries unrecognised at the time of operation*

Unfortunately, the majority of injuries are nowadays afflicted on the hepatic ducts themselves or occur high in the common hepatic duct, and it is this type of injury that may go unnoticed, particularly by a relatively inexperienced surgeon.

The common postoperative course, if such an injury occurs, is as follows—

(a)   there is a profuse discharge of bile from the wound in the early postoperative period;

(b)   intermittent fever develops;

(c)   the biliary discharge may stop and the subsequent development of either a right supra- or infra-hepatic collection of bile will require drainage;

(d)   increasing jaundice, associated with intractable pruritis, anorexia and rapid loss of weight may develop.

(e)   in many patients, after an illness associated with jaundice and intermittent fever lasting for several weeks, resolution apparently occurs, the fever abates, and the jaundice diminishes, although it seldom disappears. This is a sign that the upper end of the damaged duct or ducts is in communication with the duodenum via a fistulous tract lined by granulation tissue. Unfortunately, such tracts do not usually remain open or uninfected for very long, hence recurrent fever and jaundice can be expected after a variable interval of time.

(f)   at any time, the following serious consequences may follow the development of a stricture:

   (i)   biliary cirrhosis;
  (ii)   multiple cholangitic abscesses;
 (iii)   portal hypertension.

Determination of the level and severity of a stricture and preoperative preparation

The anatomical results of damage to the common hepatic or bile ducts and the presence or absence of a fistula can be determined by performing either a percutaneous transhepatic cholangiogram, using a Chiba needle and, if possible, endoscopic retrograde cholangiography.

These investigations having been performed, the general condition of the patient must be considered with particular regard to the state of nutrition and the presence or absence of a prolonged clotting time. Preparation of such a patient, therefore, for surgery will involve the administration of Vitamin K1, Phytomenadione BP, 15 mg daily by intramuscular injection until the prothrombin time, if prolonged, has fallen to a normal value. In addition, if the patient is extremely emaciated preoperative intravenous feeding should be considered. Adequate information should also be obtained regarding the functional capacity of the liver.

Technical principles of operative repair

Two surgeons who have been particularly associated with improvements in the management of the damaged common duct are the late Catell of the Lahey Clinic of Boston, USA, and Lord Smith, past president of the R.C.S. of St George's Hospital, London.

1   *The Catell technique*

Catell maintained, as indeed is correct, that a stricture of the ductal system can be satisfactorily repaired only if, following excision of the stricture, the proximal and distal ends of the common duct are identified and so adequately mobilised that a mucosa to mucosa anastomosis can be performed. Such a surgical technique involves prolonged and delicate dissection in an area in which almost impenetrable fibrous tissue has usually developed. Matters of technical importance when isolating the distal segment, upon which Catell laid great stress were—

(a) Reflection of the hepatic flexure in a downward and medial direction.

(b) 'Kocherisation' of the duodenum. This medial and forward mobilisation of the duodenal loop brings to the attention of the operator the common duct lymph node, which is always enlarged in such cases. This is the landmark from which the undilated lower segment of the duct can always be identified since the node lies immediately behind the duct just above the upper border of the duodenum.

(c) The mobilisation of the duodenum always reveals any fistulous communication between the upper segment and the duodenum, and this is divided. It is from this point onwards that the upward dissection towards the hilum of the liver is made in an attempt to obtain a length of undamaged hepatic duct which can then be successfully anastomosed to the isolated lower segment.

Such a repair by direct anastomosis between the two parts of the duct was always practicable when the common duct had been damaged at a relatively low level, as for example, in the classic 'tenting' injury. This repair, however, is impossible in the commoner higher injuries that occur at the present time when the hepatic duct has been damaged in the region of the porta hepatitis.

In such patients the only possible reconstructive procedure is hepaticojejunostomy, in which the short upper segment of the common duct is isolated, if necessary by splitting the hilum of the liver, and either a jejunal or Roux loop brought up to the duct and a single layer anastomosis performed. When the latter technique is used an enteroanastomosis is required several inches below the hepaticojejunal anastomosis.

Such anastomoses are difficult to perform, and in the few patients dealt with by the author he was often in doubt that a true mocosa to mucosa anastomosis had been obtained. If mucosal apposition is not achieved recurrent stricture is inevitable.

2 The Smith technique

The technique evolved by Lord Smith has greatly simplified the problem in as much as attempts at direct suture of mucosa to mucosa have been abandoned. The essential steps in the repair as performed by Lord Smith are as follows—

(a) The hepatic flexure is dissected free and displaced in a downward and medial direction (Fig. 2.8A).

(b) The dilated proximal end of the common hepatic duct is identified by probing with a needle and, once recognised, the intervening tissue is divided, the lower end of the duct being left untouched (Fig. 2.8B).

(c) A Roux loop is constructed, the end of which is closed (Fig. 2.8C).

(d) Attention is now paid to the proximal end of the duct. Through it a probe is passed upwards along the duct and then through the substance of the liver until it emerges on the surface.

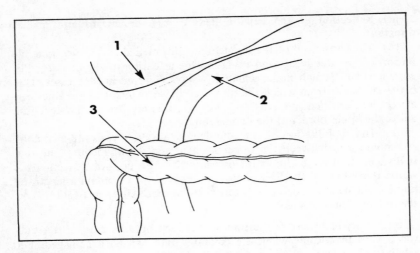

Fig 2.8 (A)   The Smith repair of biliary tract injury
1. Undersurface of liver   2. Duodenum adherant to porta hepatis   3. Hepatic flexure
reflected downwards to expose stricture and possible fistula

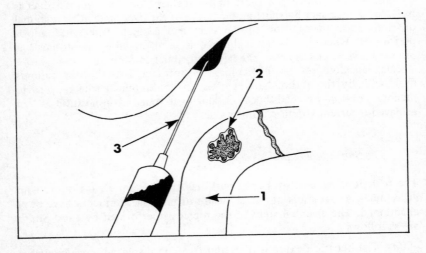

Fig 2.8 (B)
1. Duodenum separated from liver   2. Duodenal fistula opening   3. Needle aspiration
of bile from stump of common hepatic duct

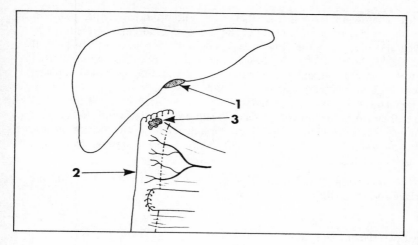

Fig 2.8 (C)
1. Opening of common hepatic or hepatic ducts above level of stricture   2. Roux loop
3. Pouting mucosa through incision made at apex of loop

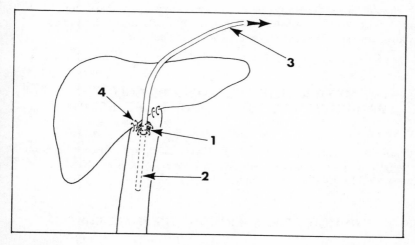

Fig 2.8 (D)
1. Mucosa sutured to suitable catheter   2. Catheter leading into Roux loop   3. Catheter
brought out through major intrahepatic duct – through liver to skin surface. Traction
impacts mucosa of jejunum against mucosa of hepatic duct   4. Buttressing sutures between
serosa of jejunum and capsule of liver

(e) The Roux loop is then held up and, proximal to the point of closure, a small incision is made in the serosa and muscular layers through which the mucosa pouts (Fig. 2.8D). The muscular layer is then pierced and a small-bore catheter is threaded into the loop. A stitch is inserted between the mucosa and the catheter so that the mucosa is held in place, after which the catheter is attached to the probe.

(f) The probe is then pulled through the substance of the liver until the catheter emerges on the surface. Pressure is exerted until the mucosal bud of the Roux loop appears to be impacted in the orifice of the common duct, after which a few reinforcing stitches between the serosa of the bowel and the liver capsule are inserted.

The operation is completed by bringing the catheter out onto the surface and then closing the abdomen.

Postoperative management

Postoperatively the catheter is syringed through, once weekly, with sterile saline to prevent the accretion of bile salts and pigment (Fig. 2.8D), and at the end of six months it is withdrawn. Lord Smith claims that this technique is successful in 95 per cent of patients, and should this prove to be true when the operation is performed elsewhere it would seem that the major problems of the damaged common bile duct have been solved.

It should, however, always be remembered that the primary aim of the surgeon is to avoid a disaster that frequently leads to a long period of invalidism and suffering before cure is eventually achieved.

2.5   THE METABOLIC CONSEQUENCES AND MANAGEMENT OF SMALL–BOWEL RESECTION

Metabolic disorders may follow small-bowel resection or disease because the length of bowel resected or diseased may be greater than can be compensated for by the remaining healthy gut.

LENGTH AND ABSORPTIVE SURFACE OF THE SMALL BOWEL

The total length of the small bowel is difficult to determine with accuracy because of the tone of the intrinsic muscles. At autopsy, in the adult it usually measures about 7 to 8 m in length, but this is an overestimate of its length in life since measurements made by means of indwelling radio-opaque intestinal tubes suggest that it may be only about 3 m long. However, the convolutions of the bowel permit it to be about 20 times as long as its mesenteric attachment.

The surface area of the gut, which determines its metabolic potential, is increased by—

(*a*) the circular folds of the mucosal surface, which begin in the second part of the duodenum and increase in number to reach their maximum in the jejunum; they diminish in frequency in the ileum and become sparse near its termination.

(*b*) each fold is covered by villi, finger-like processes of mucosa 1 mm long which project into the lumen of the gut.

(*c*) the epithelial surface of the villi is composed largely of columnar absorptive cells with a brush border consisting of tiny microvilli, which average 1 μm in length and 0.1 μm in width.

As a result of these various features it is generally conceded that, regardless of the actual length, the active surface area of the small bowel is between 20 and 40 m^2.

It should also be noted that the small intestinal mucosa has a rapid cellular turnover which leads to the replacement of the entire mucosa every two to four days, the proliferating cells being situated in the bases of the crypts.

EXTENT OF RESECTION REQUIRED TO PRODUCE DEFECTIVE FUNCTION

There can be no definite statement as to the length of the small intestine that must be removed or totally diseased before symptoms are caused. However, it can be stated that resection of the ileum, which is not only the commonest site of small bowel disease but that likely to be strangulated in an external hernia, is of greater importance than resection of the jejunum. This, despite the fact that the jejunum has taller villi and a greater absorptive area than the ileum, and that its epithelium is better endowed with enzymes, thus producing comparatively greater chemical and absorptive capacity. Resection of as little as 125 cm of ileum may, in the author's experience, lead to persistent diarrhoea even though the actual presence of overt steatorrhoea cannot be identified. Normal fat absorption can be maintained when as little as 40 cm of ileum remains, but with a lesser length than this steatorrhoea is common.

The relatively greater importance of the ileum is probably due to the following factors—

(*a*) the more rapid transit of intestinal contents after a distal resection;
(*b*) the jejunum being less adaptive than the ileum;
(*c*) abnormal bacterial flora developing in the remaining gut;
(*d*) ileal resection leads to severe disturbances of bile salt metabolism.

After ileal resection there is a diminution of the bile salt pool because of a disruption of bile salt resorption. There eventually follows a decrease in the jejunal concentration of bile salts and a fall in the incorporation of lipids into the micellar phase. This decreases fat absorption and as a result steatorrhoea follows. Since a reduction in fat absorption is accompanied by decreased absorption of fat soluble vitamins, vitamin D, vitamin B_{12} and folic acid deficiency develops, the first associated with tetany and the latter with megaloblastic anaemia.

COMPENSATORY CHANGES FOLLOWING MASSIVE RESECTION

Resection is followed by compensatory functional and structural changes in the remaining bowel. Animal experiments in the rat, however, have shown that whereas resection of the jejunum causes a marked enlargement of the ileum, the converse does not occur. Microscopic hyperplasia of the villi follows resection of either jejunum or ileum, although changes in the latter are always more obvious. Villous height is known to increase very rapidly following a proximal resection, the probable stimulus being the amount of nutrient presented to the remaining bowel. In animals, it has been shown that the anatomical changes following resection are mirrored by an increase in function of the remaining bowel. However, in man, the results are very variable. Some data in the literature suggests that the improvement in absorptive capacity may not necessarily be the same for all measurable parameters. Thus, fat absorption may improve while amino-acid absorption remains poor.

CHIEF CAUSES OF SMALL BOWEL RESECTION

The common causes of small gut resection include—

1 Resection of non-viable gut following strangulation by bands, internal or external herniae.
2 Strictures caused by—
   (a) fibrosis, as in the intestinal stenosis of Garré;
   (b) inflammation, tuberculosis or Crohn's disease;
   (c) malignant, adenocarcinoma or carcinoid tumours.
3 Diverticulosis of the small bowel, following perforation.
4 Intestinal infarction caused by mesenteric thrombosis or embolus.
5 Volvulus, particularly in the neonate.

Of these various causes, mesenteric thrombosis affecting the superior mesenteric artery, or volvulus of the midgut, are the most serious since both are associated with massive resection involving the whole of the small bowel from a point just distal to the duodenojejunal flexure to the junction of the mid and lateral third of the transverse colon. However, Crohn's disease may cause equal difficulties because functional deterioration takes place even in the absence of a demonstrable mucosal lesion.

EFFECTS OF MASSIVE RESECTION

Massive jejunoileal resection is followed by three phases—

1 In the early postoperative period, once intestinal motility has returned, there is an excessive loss of fluid and electrolytes which may amount to several litres daily, and the severity of the ensuing diarrhoea may cause tenesmus and severe perianal excoriation and pain. The factors precipitating such a massive outpouring of fluid include—

(a)   total failure of absorption of food or fluid administered orally;
(b)   hyperacidity of the bowel contents;
(c)   defective absorption of the bile salts which on entering the large bowel cause mucosal irritation and the retention of water, with the production of the so-called cholereiform diarrhoea;
(d)   decreased transit time.

2 In the intermediate phase, the phase of adaptation, the severe diarrhoea improves but the body weight falls and attention must be focused on the nutritional disturbance.

3 In the final phase, a balance is achieved between the absorptive capacity of the bowel and the degree of physical activity.

A review of the literature suggests that approximately a third of the small bowel can be resected without the development of a severe metabolic disturbance. In an animal such as the dog, survival is possible after an 80 per cent resection so long as the diet is strictly controlled. In general, nutritional balance studies in the human confirm that after massive resections the absorption of fat, together with fat soluble vitamins, is severely disturbed, protein absorption is moderately decreased, but the utilisation of carbohydrate remains fairly normal.

CHIEF METABOLIC CONSEQUENCES OF RESECTION

1   Diminished fat absorption

Diminished fat absorption causes steatorrhoea, the frequent passage of bulky, offensive stools being a distressing experience to the patient. The major site of fat absorption is the duodenum and proximal jejunum, absorption being completed within 100 cm of the duodenojejunal junction. Paradoxically, however, a resection of the distal ileum causes much greater diminution in fat absorption because of the disturbance it produces in the enterohepatic circulation of the bile salts. These may be considered as detergents, the steroid nucleus being lipid soluble and the hydroxyl groups water soluble. At high concentrations, bile salts form spherical polymolecular aggregates (micelles) the lipid soluble parts of each molecule being orientated towards the centre. As the bile salt concentration rises to a critical level, so micelles composed of cholesterol, fat soluble vitamins, fatty acid and monoglycerides are formed, and are absorbed. However, the total bile salt pool in man is only 2 to 4 g and 99 per cent of this is within the enterohepatic circulation. It is estimated that the liver secretes 20 to 30 g of bile salts a day into the intestine, six to eight times the total pool. Only 15 to 20 per cent of the total is lost daily, representing a 3 to 4 per cent loss with each cycle. The hepatic production of new bile salts, replenishing that which is lost, is approximately 0.8 g daily. It has been shown that an ileal resection of greater length than 50 cm will lead to a fall in the intestinal concentration of bile salts and that a reduction of the enterohepatic circulation of bile salts by some 20 per cent represents the maximal adaptive ability of the liver to make up for the loss.

Other factors that increase the severity of the steatorrhoea are—

(a) the colonisation of the bowel by organisms which deconjugate the bile salts, thus reducing the critical micellar concentration. These organisms include the bacteriodes, *Streptococcus faecalis,* and *Clostridium perfringens.* Logically, it would seem reasonable to replace the missing bile salts by a mixture of sodium taurocholate and sodium glycocholate but, unfortunately, although this may reduce the actual steatorrhoea it does not necessarily add to the patient's comfort since a spill-over of a proportion of the unabsorbed bile acid into the colon produces a cathartic effect because of the inhibition of water and salt absorption. As a result, large volumes of fluid faeces may replace the bulky motions of steatorrhoea.

Thus, the paradox of the clinical situation arises in that patients may feel better and have fewer bowel actions if the already depleted bile salt pool is depleted still further by the administration of drugs such as cholestyramine, which is an ion exchange resin that binds bile acids in the intestinal lumen and thus prevents their cathartic effect.

(b) inactivation of lipase by the high pH in the small bowel.

2   Duodenal ulceration

The high pH in the small intestine causes a further potentially disastrous effect in that the hormone gastrin, normally secreted by the cells of the pyloric antrum, is not inhibited. In consequence, gastric secretion continues at a high level and duodenal ulceration commonly complicates small bowel resection. Previously, this complication was often so severe that gastric surgery was required, but it is now possible that the continuous administration of the drug cimetidine may be capable of controlling this undesirable side effect.

Other metabolic effects of intestinal inadequacy include—

Megaloblastic anaemia

The gradual development of megaloblastic anaemia due to the defective absorption of vitamin B_{12} and folic acid may be simply the result of an ileal resection or, if the resection has been associated with the production of blind loops, e.g. a side-to-side anastomosis, bacterial contamination will reinforce the effect. Less commonly, the vitamin deficiency is caused by extensive mucosal disease.

Folic acid is somewhat different from vitamin B_{12} in that neither intrinsic factor nor any other substance is necessary for its absorption and, furthermore, it is absorbed over wide areas of the small intestine, particularly the jejunum. However, a vitamin B_{12} deficiency will become obvious only when the body's store has been exhausted, the normal liver containing approximately three year's supply.

The clinical effects of vitamin B_{12} deficiency include—

(a) Glossitis: when acute the tongue is red, painful and ulcerated. More commonly it is smooth, atrophic and sore.
(b) Jaundice: when the anaemia becomes severe there may be slight jaundice giving rise to the typical lemon yellow colour of the skin.
(c) Hepatomegaly: due to fatty infiltration of the liver.
(d) In five to ten per cent of patients a neuropathy develops that usually begins in the lower limbs. The sensory loss is of a glove-and-stocking type and is accompanied by loss of the deep tendon reflexes. Extension of the neuropathy to the spinal cord results in loss of vibration sense and proprioception and, finally, when the disease extends to the lateral columns a spastic paraparesis occurs.

The diagnosis of macrocytic anaemia is confirmed by the following laboratory findings—

(a) reduction in haemoglobin concentration;
(b) macrocytosis;
(c) a normal mean corpuscular haemoglobin concentration associated with variation in size and shape of the red cell;
(d) bone marrow aspiration indicates an abnormal pattern of megaloblastic erythropoiesis;
(e) serum vitamin B_{12} level is less than 100 pg/100 ml.

Magnesium and calcium deficiency

The clinical manifestations caused by magnesium deficiency are related to a number of factors which include—

(a) the availability of the ion;
(b) the concentration of other ions, notably calcium;
(c) the pH of the plasma.

The actual amount of magnesium present in the extracellular fluid is insignificant as far as the osmolality-maintaining function is concerned. The chief role of magnesium is in regulating enzymatic activity and neuro-muscular excitability.

Thus, the symptoms and signs of hypomagnesaemia are those of central nervous and neuromuscular hyperactivity. The deep tendon reflexes are exaggerated, fasciculation occurs in the muscles, tremor, and personality changes may be observed. Both Trousseau's and Chvostek's signs are positive, and convulsions have been reported. The symptoms and signs, therefore, closely resemble those associated with hypocalcaemia but the serum calcium would be found to be normal if the hypomagnesaemia existed alone. However, in patients suffering from massive resection of the bowel, accompanying hypocalcaemia is also common. The symptoms of hypomagnesaemia can often be relieved, if only temporarily, by the administration of calcium, but the calcium levels return to normal only after the simultaneous administration of magnesium.

The diagnosis of magnesium deficiency is confirmed in the laboratory. Serum plasma levels may be low but are not reliable. More importance should be placed on a diminished concentration of this ion in the red cells, normally 5.3 ± 0.53 mEq/mmol/litre and a diminished urine secretion, less than 2 mEq/mmol/24 hours.

Hypoalbuminaemia

It appears from the literature that the absorption of protein is less affected than fat. Nevertheless, following a massive resection, excessive nitrogen loss occurs in the stools mainly in the form of undigested meat fibres. The level to which the plasma proteins fall varies according to the length of the resection. In one case reported, in which only 8 inches of jejunum remained, the serum proteins fell progressively to 20 g/litre albumin and 24 g/litre globulin, and gross oedema developed. These changes were accompanied by a fatty degeneration of the liver similar to that observed in famine.

Sugar absorption

Massive resection results in a glucose tolerance curve that is flat and slow to rise. Similarly, D-xylose absorption, which is commonly used as a test of upper jejunal function, becomes grossly abnormal. Normally, following an oral dose of 25 g, more than 4.5 g should be recovered from the urine in the next 5 hours.

Gastric hypersecretion

Note has already been made of the possible development of severe duodenal ulceration following massive resection.

Cholereiform diarrhoea

The failure to absorb bile salts and their consequent overspill into the colon precipitates watery diarrhoea. This is apparently more marked in the morning, due to the accumulation of bile salts in the colon during the night. A further factor may be the irritant effects of unabsorbed soaps and fatty acids in the intestinal lumen.

Gall-stone formation

A two- to threefold increase in gall-stone formation has been reported in patients subjected to small-bowel resection, which is again attributed to the disturbed enterohepatic circulation of bile salts. In theory, if the bile salts decrease in quantity the relative concentration in the bile should fall, disturbing cholesterol solubilisation and producing a lithogenic bile. In practice, this appears to happen, although the experimental evidence is somewhat conflicting because, in the Rhesus monkey, while the concentration of bile salts falls the phospholipid concentration rises. Such a change would tend to overcome the adverse effects of the falling bile acid concentration because lecithin associates with the cholesterol fraction to form a liquid crystalline phase.

TREATMENT

The treatment of patients who have undergone massive resection is difficult. The initial resection, which is usually performed in the presence of massive intestinal gangrene, carries a high immediate mortality, following which, in the presence of only a limited intestinal capacity, death occurs in many patients within a few months. The critical bowel length appears to be in the region of 35 to 40 cm. The introduction of intravenous amino acids and fat emulsion may, however, make a significant difference to t' ⨼ immediate results although no comprehensive reports have yet appeared in the literature showing whether or not these preparations have made a significant impact on the *late* results.

Initial treatment

Most observers are agreed that it is in the first few weeks, during the period of intense diarrhoea, that care should be taken to monitor the rapidly changing levels of serum electrolytes, and it may be assumed that rapid loss of body weight which has been previously reported would now be partially, if not wholly, controlled by the use of intravenous amino acid and lipid preparations.

Later treatment

1   *Diet*

There is considerable evidence that fat may be replaced by medium chain triglycerides with a consequent decrease in the degree of steatorrhoea, but if such replacement is complete the diet becomes unpalatable. However, when the total fat in the diet is reduced the faecal fat excretion falls and this reduces the diarrhoea but if this is done at the same time it diminishes the total amount of fat absorbed.

Calories. A high calorie diet should be provided containing up to 3000 kcal. It should be high in carbohydrate and high or medium in protein. Starches should be avoided because they lead to increased intestinal fermentation, causing cramps and abdominal distension.

2   *Drug therapy*

(*a*)   Since the transit time through the gastrointestinal tract may be as little as 5 minutes, drugs which control peristaltic activity may be helpful. These include diphenoxylate hydrochloride or, alternatively, codeine phosphate.

(*b*)   Cholestyramine. The use of this drug has already been discussed. Essentially it is a resin capable of binding bile salts and, therefore, will remove their cathartic effect on the colon. However, if the bile salts are removed, an attempt must be made to replace their micellar activity by materials that will aid fat absorption without irritating the colon. One such compound is Polysorbate 80. This is a mixture of oleic esters of sorbitol which substances are able to produce stable emulsions that are but little affected by high concentrations of electrolytes or intestinal pH.

(*c*)   The fat soluble vitamins A, B_{12}, D and K should be given to prevent the corresponding vitamin deficiency syndrome.

3   *Surgical treatment*

(*a*)   Severe duodenal ulceration developing from the hyperchlorhydria may require vagotomy if it cannot be controlled by drugs such as cimetidine.

(*b*)   The reversed intestinal loop. Although there is considerable experimental evidence, chiefly in the dog and rat, that reversed segments decrease weight loss after massive resection and cause an improvement in fat absorption, there are comparatively few studies in the human, and little is known of the optimum length which such a reversed loop should measure; lengths of between 7.5 cm and 10 cm have been suggested.

2.6   TUMOURS OF THE LARGE BOWEL, AETIOLOGY, PATHOLOGY, SYMPTOMATOLOGY AND TREATMENT

Incidence

In Western society, between 9 and 20 per cent of all deaths from cancer are due to colorectal neoplasms. However, even in the industrialised nations their incidence varies considerably being, for example, three times greater in Scotland than in Finland. Furthermore, within the Western countries themselves there remains a marked difference between rural and urban communities, a significantly lower incidence occurring in the former.

Causation

(*a*)   *Hereditary factors*

In a small minority of patients the underlying cause of a colorectal cancer is immediately obvious. Thus, patients suffering from familial polyposis, Gardner's or Turcot's syndrome inevitably develop carcinoma of the large bowel or rectum.

(*b*)   *Dietary factors*

In the majority of patients, however, the underlying cause is not immediately apparent although in the last two decades epidemiological studies have led to the suggestion that the most likely cause of large bowel cancer is a dietary fault. This hypothesis is supported by the fact that carcinoma of the large bowel is more frequent in the higher socio-economic groups and that in those non-Western societies that have adopted a Western type of diet a greater incidence of colorectal cancer has developed.

The extraneous dietary factors that have been blamed are too high an intake of protein, carbohydrate and fat, combined with a diminished intake of fibre.

(c)   Bacteriological factors

However, the hypothesis which has gained most acceptance at the present time is that colonic cancer is caused by the interaction of the requirements for or the products of digestion and the intestinal bacteria. So far as the latter are concerned it has been shown that the number of anaerobic Bacteriodes present in the gut varies with the incidence of colorectal cancer; their numbers being smaller in the less prone and higher in the faeces of high risk populations. The mode of action of these organisms lies in the degradation of bile acid cholate to the potentially carcinogenic deoxycholate and their importance has been experimentally demonstrated by the finding that carcinogens which will induce tumours in normal rats fail to do so in a sterile environment.

(d)   Fibre intake

The importance of fibre intake lies in the reduction of faecal bulk which follows decreased intake which in turn is followed by a greatly increased faecal transit time, thus allowing greater exposure of the colonic mucosa to any carcinogenic agent present in the lumen. The daily dry weight of the faeces of the rural black African is between 40 and 70 g compared to an average of 20–25 g for the dry weight of the faeces of the urban white. In the former the faeces are voluminous, soft and passed with ease whereas in the latter the faeces are usually small, segmented and hard. In the former the transit time is low, 10 hours, in the latter high, between 24 to 28 hours.

PATHOLOGY OF COLONIC TUMOURS

1   Polyps

A polyp is defined as an outgrowth from the mucosal surface.

(a) *Juvenile polyps.* Technically, these are probably hamartomata, i.e. tumour-like malformations in which the tissues of a particular part of the body are arranged haphazardly, usually with an excess of one or more of its components. Such lesions have no tendency to grow excessively and usually stop growing after puberty. In the colon, 70 per cent form solitary tumours which are nearly always pedunculated. Their peak incidence is about 5 years of age. The common presenting symptoms are:

   (i)   rectal bleeding,
   (ii)   prolapse through the anus,
   (iii) they may cause recurrent rectal prolapse.

(b) *Sessile polyps.* These are the commonest 'tumours' of the large bowel and the majority are caused by benign hyperplasia without structural evidence of neoplastic change. They form smoothly rounded elevations above the normal mucosa 1 to 5 mm in diameter. Microscopic examination demonstrates a degree of cellular hyperplasia accompanied by differentiation into absorptive and goblet cells. The source of the increased cellular division which finally leads to polyp formation is the proliferative portion of the crypts of Lieberkühn.

(c) *Adenomatous polyps* (pedunculated adenoma). By definition an adenoma is a simple tumour of solid glandular tissue consisting of a dense mass of acini lined by exuberant epithelium. Adenomata arising in glands opening directly on to a surface often become pedunculated. Proximal to the sigmoid colon adenomata are relatively rare; 70 per cent are located in the rectum, rectosigmoid, or lower sigmoid, 20 per cent in the proximal sigmoid, and only 10 per cent in the remaining colon.

(a) *Macroscopic appearance*

Adenomatous polyps are usually less than 2 cm in diameter and form spherical or hemispherical excrescences with a head attached to the colon by a stalk. The latter is normally covered by normal looking colonic mucosa and has an inner core of connective tissue which arises from the submucosa. The head of the polyp varies in size from 0.3 to 5 cm and is usually pink to red in colour. The surface is smooth or mamillated.

(b) *Histological structure*

Microscopic examination shows a histological appearance varying between a fairly normal colonic pattern to a picture of elongated hyperplastic glands. Atypical cells, sufficiently abnormal to be classified as carcinoma in situ, may be present but if such cancerous changes do not invade the stalk, cure is effected by removal of the polyp. The incidence of true invasive malignancy in adenomatous polyps is probably not greater than 5 per cent and is exceptional in tumours of this type when they are less than 1.5 cm in diameter, but somewhat commoner in tumours larger than this.

Specific syndromes associated with pedunculated adenoma are familial polyposis, Gardner's syndrome and Turcot's syndrome.

Familial polyposis

This rare condition is an autosomal dominant trait so that if one parent is affected half the children will inherit the disease but only those that are affected will transmit the disease. This has three stages; at birth and during early childhood there are neither symptoms nor signs and sigmoidoscopy is negative. In adolescence and early adult life polyps gradually appear and during the second and third decades diarrhoea begins and malignant degeneration of the polyps occurs. The polyps range in size from 0.5 to 5 cm in diameter and carpet the whole of the colonic mucosa although they are most common in the distal colon and rectum. If no polyps have appeared by 40 years of age the offending gene is absent.

Gardner's syndrome

This condition is also transmitted as an autosomal dominant trait and resembles polyposis coli. However, there are additional features in the form of osteomata and soft tissue malformations. The former occur in the mandible, orbit, calvarium, pelvis and long bones. The latter may take the form of desmoid tumours occurring in surgical scars or within the peritoneal cavity, sebaceous cysts, or multiple lipomata. Such skeletal and soft tissue abnormalities sometimes develop prior to the appearance of the polyps.

Turcot's syndrome

A syndrome transmitted as an autosomal recessive characterised by the development of colonic polyps and neurological tumours.

2   Villous sessile adenomata

These are relatively rare and comprise only 10 per cent of all benign lesions of the colon. Commonly single, they are papillary tumours attached to the colon by a broad base often extending over wide areas of the mucosal surface. They are most frequently found in the rectum and sigmoid. Microscopically, villous tumours are composed of finger-like papillary villi which may branch. This tumour has a significant potential for malignant transformation, estimated by Morson of St Mark's Hospital to be as high as 40 per cent.

3   Primary malignant tumours of the colon

The gross morphological features of colonic primary adenocarcinoma are variable and have considerable influence on the symptomatology of the disease. They are described as: polypoidal, nodular, ulcerating, scirrhous and colloid.

(a)   Microscopical features

Colonic carcinomata, according to their degree of differentiation, resemble the tissue of origin. In well-differentiated tumours the neoplastic cells are grouped in acinar-like clusters simulating normal glands, whereas in poorly differentiated or anaplastic tumours, cells with little resemblance to colonic mucosal cells are dispersed in irregular sheets or cords with no suggestion of glandular formation.

(b)   Relation of site to macroscopic type

In general, tumours on the right side of the colon tend to be polypoidal, and to ulcerate later, whereas on the left side tumours tend to be infiltrative, scirrhous, annular and circumferential which results in the tumour being' intramural rather than intraluminal and in consequence infiltrating and thickening the bowel wall.

(c)   Distribution of colorectal neoplasms

The distribution of large bowel tumours is as follows—

Caecum 10 per cent
Ascending colon 8 per cent
Transverse colon 12 per cent
Descending colon 6 per cent
Sigmoid colon 26 per cent
Rectum 28 per cent
Multiple tumours occur in 3 to 4 per cent.

(d)   Tumour spread

   (i)   Locally in the bowel wall both in a vertical direction and to the peritoneal surface;
   (ii)   by the lymphatics: lymphatic spread occurs via the lymph vessels of the bowel wall to related lymph nodes—in the proximal part of the large intestine, lymph nodes are especially numerous in the mesocolon and adjacent retroperitoneal tissues;
   (iii) by the venous system to the liver;
   (iv)   transcoelomic spread: gravitational metastases may occur at any time after the tumour has penetrated the bowel to involve the serosal surface, after which cells may be detached and seeded in the peritoneal cavity. Such seedling deposits eventually result in a shelf of malignant tissue developing in the pouch of Douglas or, in women, secondary deposits in the ovaries which are known as Krukenberg tumours.

(e)   Staging

The classical description of staging carcinoma of the colon is that described by Dukes—

Stage A: A lesion confined to the mucosa.
Stage B_1:   A lesion extending into but not through the muscularis mucosae; lymph node negative.
Stage B_2:   A lesion penetrating the muscularis mucosae; lymph node negative.
Stage C_1:   A lesion limited to the wall; paracolic lymph nodes positive.
Stage C_2:   A lesion involving all layers; lymph nodes positive to highest point of ligature.

Duke's staging gives a reliable indication of survival (Fig. 2.9), and it is of interest to note that the mortality statistics for carcinoma of the colon have remained depressingly constant over the past 25 years.

SYMPTOMS ASSOCIATED WITH COLONIC TUMOURS

Right-sided tumours

The symptoms associated with tumours of the right colon are determined by—

(i)   the gross pathological features of tumours in this area; the majority of tumours in this segment of the colon tend to be polypoidal and ulcerating;
(ii) the liquidity of the faecal stream;
(iii) the large calibre and distensibility of the right colon.

Thus, with the exception of tumours situated in the region adjacent to the ileo-caecal valve, tumours in the ascending and transverse colon rarely cause intestinal obstruction. The more common symptoms are—

(a) vague abdominal pain, 80 per cent;
(b) general malaise and lassitude associated with anaemia, 20 per cent.
(c) a palpable abdominal mass, 67 per cent;
(d) symptoms and signs suggesting the development of an appendix mass—this is particularly common if subacute perforation occurs or should the tumour act as the obstructing agent to the appendix itself, 20 per cent;
(e) when the tumour is situated at the hepatic flexure, or the caecum has failed to descend, it is possible to mistake a perforating carcinoma for acute cholecystitis.
(f) melaena, 8 per cent;
(g) weight loss, 48 per cent.

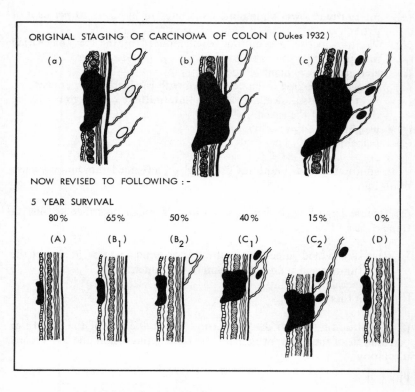

Fig 2.9   Original staging of carcinoma of colon (Dukes 1932)
(a)   Tumour limited to wall of rectum
(b)   Tumour extending to extra rectal tissues but no evidence of lymphatic spread
(c)   Tumour associated with metastatic spread
            Now revised to following
(A)   Tumour confined to mucosa
(B_1)   Tumour extending to but not through the muscularis mucosa
(B_2)   Tumour penetrating the muscularis mucosa – Lymph nodes negative
(C_1)   Tumour limited to wall of bowel plus paracolic lymph node involvement
(C_2)   Tumour together with lymph node involvement to highest point of ligature
(D)   Local condition unimportant. Distant metastases present

Left-sided tumours

Due to the frequency with which tumours of the descending colon tend to be circumferential and because the faeces are semisolid, the common symptoms associated with left-sided growths are—

(*a*) intermittent lower abdominal colic, present in 50 to 70 per cent of patients;
(*b*) loss of appetite, a symptom often induced by the fear that eating may precipitate the onset of pain;
(*c*) change in bowel habit, 60 per cent;
(*d*) recognisable blood intimately mixed with the faeces, 10 per cent;
(*e*) right iliac fossa swelling, due to intermittent obstruction causing distension of the caecum;
(*f*) weight loss, 14 per cent;
(*g*) palpable mass, 45 per cent.

In addition to the symptoms listed above, left-sided tumours may also result in—

(*a*) acute large bowel obstruction which is usually ascribed to one of three causes:

  (i) superadded infection resulting in a rapid increase in size of the tumour and sudden occlusion of the lumen;
  (ii) faecal impaction;
  (iii) intussusception.

(*b*) Peritonitis. This is due to perforation at the site of the growth or perforation of the bowel proximal to an obstructing lesion due to stercoral ulceration.

Physical signs associated with colonic carcinoma

(*a*) A palpable mass is most commonly associated with right-sided tumours, a tumour in this situation being palable in approximately 50 to 75 per cent of patients compared with only some 30 to 45 per cent of patients suffering from tumours of the descending colon. Lesions of the sigmoid colon may be palpable per rectum as an extra rectal mass.

(*b*) Anaemia. This is normocytic and hypochromic and associated with a low serum iron. A history of failure of such anaemia to improve following the administration of oral iron therapy is relatively common.

(*c*) Abdominal distension and borborygmi if chronic large bowel obstruction is present.

(*d*)   Signs of local or general peritonitis will follow perforation of the tumour or a stercoral ulcer if obstruction should occur.

INVESTIGATION

(*a*)   Sigmoidoscopy and biopsy

Because approximatley 50 per cent of colorectal cancers occur within the terminal 25 cm of the large bowel, inclusive of the rectum, sigmoidoscopy is mandatory. It should be performed, if possible, without any preliminary bowel preparation since even when the tumour itself cannot be seen the character of the contents of the bowel may be very suggestive of a lesion at a higher level. When a lesion is seen, a biopsy should be taken to establish the precise pathology of the lesion. The differential diagnosis of carcinoma of the lower sigmoid includes proctocolitis, large bowel Crohn's disease, amoebic dysentery, and benign or malignant villous papilloma.

The common appearance of a visible lesion is one of an ulcer surrounded by an edge that is everted and the base of which is commonly greyish in colour. Less commonly, colloid cancers form large soft, friable, gelatinous ulcerating tumours which may produce mucous in such large quantities that the lesion cannot be distinguished from the papillary type of adenocarcinoma; the malignant counterpart of the villous papilloma.

(*b*)   Barium enema

When sigmoidoscopy is negative, a barium enema is the next logical investigation. The accuracy of this examination has been greatly increased by the introduction of double contrast techniques by which the radiologist is able to demonstrate lesions in areas which are difficult to visualise, such as the overlapping parts of the sigmoid colon. Lesions of the caecum are also better delineated and polyps can usually be distinguished from faecal masses.

The radiological appearance of a carcinoma of the colon depends upon its site and its type. Classically, the common ulcerating tumour causes a filling defect with a typical fingerprint deformity or 'shouldering' at its margins. The more scirrhous types of tumour may cause an annular constricting lesion extending for a variable distance along the bowel to produce the characteristic 'napkin-ring' appearance. Both types are associated with mucosal destruction at the site of the lesion.

(*c*)   Colonoscopy

In centres suitably equipped with both instrumentation and expertise it is now possible to supplement the investigations described by colonoscopy. This is indicated particularly if:

(i)   the diagnosis remains uncertain following barium enema;

(ii)   the lesion demonstrated by the barium enema is a polyp, since colonoscopic resection of these tumours has now virtually replaced open laparotomy.

(d)   Haematological examination

There are no specific haematological tests to enable a distinction to be drawn between the various causes of diarrhoea, but since any case of blood loss will eventually result in anaemia, the haemoglobin and red cell count should be determined in order that the anaemia, if found, can be corrected before operation. In tumours of the right colon an anaemia refractory to iron is a highly suggestive feature of the disease.

(e)   Tumour markers

The colorectal tumour antigen first described in 1965 was initially believed to be specific for malignant tumours of the colon and rectum, but it was also known to be a component of embryonic colon tissue and for this reason was named the carcinoembryonic antigen or CEA. This nomenclature is now regarded as incorrect, further investigation having shown that the same antigen is present in normal serum, in normal adult colon tissue, and other gastrointestinal cancers. The more correct terminology is oncofetal antigen, i.e. an antigen associated with both fetal material and tumour tissue, perhaps because both are composed of rapidly growing cells.

An estimation of CEA is of little value in the initial diagnosis but is of some value as an indicator of metastatic recurrence since elevation to above normal values occurs in the presence of hepatic metastases. Furthermore, it has been shown that the level of CEA tends to rise above normal values in individuals who eventually develop metastatic disease following surgery.

TREATMENT OF COLONIC CANCER

Preoperative bowel preparation

In the absence of complications, or general contra-indications to surgery, the treatment of all colonic cancers is surgical resection. This must be preceded by suitable preoperative preparation one of the most important aspects of which is local preparation of the bowel itself.

The most suitable method of cleansing the bowel is still a matter for debate.

(a) The conventional method of bowel preparation consisted of a low residue diet, oral magnesium sulphate, repeated enemata and washouts.

(b) In 1975, Crapp and others described the method known as 'whole bowel irrigation' in which, on the day before operation, normal saline is infused through an indwelling nasogastric tube until the fluid passed per rectum is clear for at least 30 minutes.

Such mechanical cleansing reduces the mass of faeces so that although the number of bacteria per gram of faeces remains unchanged the total bacterial content of the colon is reduced. The efficiency of mechanical cleansing has recently been shown to be still further improved by the use of an elemental diet such as Vivonex for periods of up to a week preoperatively.

(c) The majority of surgeons would use, in addition to mechanical cleansing, antimicrobial drugs. Those commonly in use at the present time and which have been found to be highly effective, include neomycin and metronidazole, the former being particularly active against the *Escherichia coli* and the latter against *Bacteriodes fragilis,* both organisms commonly found in wound infections following colonic resection.

Controlled trials have shown that the incidence of wound infection following colonic surgery is significantly reduced by the introduction of antimicrobial drugs into the preoperative regime.

Resection

The essential operative principles underlying definitive surgery for colonic cancer are—

(a) wide removal of the cancer-bearing segment of bowel

Before proceeding with resection, the whole colon must be carefully examined to exclude the presence of a second tumour, after which the abdominal cavity as a whole is examined to determine the presence of absence of:

(i)   lymphatic metastases;
(ii) peritoneal seedlings;
(iii) hepatic metastases.

Thereafter, attention is paid to the tumour itself, noting particularly the presence of extracolonic invasion and adherence of the tumour to the abdominal wall or other viscera.

(b) wide excision of the lymphatics draining the involved segment

In general terms the lymphatics of the right and transverse colon accompany the tributaries of the superior mesenteric vein whereas those of the left colon, from the splenic flexure downwards, are associated with the tributaries of the inferior mesenteric.

(c) the performance of the resection.

This must be carried out with a minimum degree of contamination of the peritoneal cavity by both bacteria and malignant cells.

Extent of Resection

The following are the normally accepted limits of resection for tumours in various parts of the colon.

(*a*) *Carcinoma of the right colon including tumours of the hepatic flexure*

These are treated by right hemicolectomy. The terminal ileum is removed, together with the colon as far as the junction of the right two-thirds with that of the left one-third. The branches of the superior mesenteric artery. including the middle colic, right colic and inferior colic, together with the terminal branches of the ileocolic vessel itself, are ligated and divided at their junction with the main trunk.

(*b*) *Carcinoma of the transverse colon*

These are treated by excision of the whole of the transverse colon and mesocolon. The middle colic artery is divided at its origin from the superior mesenteric, and if the tumour lies at the level of the splenic flexure the ascending branch of the inferior mesenteric artery will also require division.

(*c*) *Carcinoma of the descending colon*

This is normally treated by left hemicolectomy, the left third of the transverse colon, and the descending and sigmoid colon up to the junction of the rectosigmoid junction being excised. This extensive resection involves division of the inferior mesenteric artery proximal to the origin of its branches.

(*d*) *Carcinoma of the sigmoid*

This is treated by sigmoid colectomy, the first, second and third sigmoid branches of the inferior mesenteric artery being divided close to their origin from the inferior mesenteric artery.

(*e*) *Polyposis coli*

This condition, in the absence of malignant change in any of the rectal polyps, is commonly treated by total colectomy followed by ileo-rectal anastomosis. Prior to colectomy the rectal polyps are first destroyed by diathermy, several sessions usually being required. This is performed before resection because it is relatively easier to accomplish when the faecal stream is solid.

The anastomosis

(*a*) Following right hemicolectomy, the continuity of the bowel may be restored by end-to-end, side-to-end, or side-to-side anastomosis. The potential long-term complication of the last mentioned method is the eventual development of the 'blind loop' syndrome.

(*b*) Following all other types of resection end-to-end anastomosis should be performed.

(*c*) Technique of anastomosis. Some disagreement exists as to the best method of actually performing the anastomosis and whether or not this should be carried out by single-layer inverting or everting technique, or by the standard two-layer techniques. The argument arises because anastomotic dehiscence is responsible for at least 10 per cent of deaths following colonic resections.

Comparisons have been made in both the experimental animal and the human.

(*a*) In the rabbit a single-layer inverting type of suture appears to be superior to the standard two-layer technique or the everting type of suture judged on the incidence of anastomotic dehiscence and perianastomotic leakage.

(*b*) In the human, however, randomised trials comparing single-layer and two-layer anastomoses have shown that a similar incidence of anastomotic dehiscence and obstructive complications occurs after both types of anastomosis. In addition to clinical evidence of anastomotic dehiscence, subclinical dehiscence, as judged by postoperative barium enema examination, also occurs following either technique. Thus, it would seem that a single-layer inverting anastomosis is in no way superior to the standard two-layer.

The frequency of anastomotic dehiscence appears to depend upon several factors including—

(*a*) The adequacy of bowel preparation. A significant correlation exists between faecal loading and anastomotic dehiscence.

(*b*) Faecal soiling and peritoneal sepsis can be shown in the experimental animal to impair significantly the healing of colonic anastomoses, but in the human such factors tend to be minimised by the use of broad-spectrum antibiotics.

(*c*) Nutritional status. A significant correlation exists between hypoproteinaemia and anastomotic disruption in both the experimental animal and the human.

Mortality

The immediate mortality following colonic resection, in the absence of obstruction or perforation, varies between 5 and 10 per cent according to the series examined. The major causes of death include—

(a)   anastomotic dehiscence, followed by intra-abdominal sepsis;
(b)   cardiovascular complications;
(c)   pulmonary embolus.

COMPLICATIONS OF COLONIC NEOPLASMS AND THEIR TREATMENT

The two major complications of colonic neoplasms are—

(a)   intestinal obstruction;
(b)   perforation followed by local abscess formation or general peritonitis.

The frequency of these two complications varies somewhat according to the series examined but in a group of 700 patients reviewed by the author the incidence of each was as follows—

(a)   Intestinal obstruction

This occurred in 28 per cent of patients with tumours situated in the caecum, ascending colon or hepatic flexure; 26 per cent in tumours involving the transverse colon; and 40 per cent in tumours arising from the splenic flexure, descending colon and sigmoid.

(b)   Peritonitis

This complication arises as a result of perforation of a stercoral ulcer in association with intestinal obstruction, or from perforation of the growth itself. The former nearly always results in general peritonitis whereas when perforation of the growth itself occurs a local peritonitis follows, particularly when the tumour involves the right colon.

The incidence of peritonitis in patients suffering from obstruction is remarkedly low, in this series accounting for only 1.5 per cent of all cases, the majority occurring in left-sided tumours. In non-obstructed patients the overall incidence of peritonitis was 10 per cent, general peritonitis being somewhat commoner than local. However, local peritonitis is a particular feature of caecal tumours whereas general peritonitis occurs much more frequently when the tumour involves the descending colon and sigmoid.

Treatment of the complications

1   *Intestinal obstruction*

(*a*) When the obstructing lesion is proximal to the distal third of the transverse colon a formal right hemicolectomy should be performed. The presence of a degree of small bowel dilatation is technically helpful since it increases the ease with which an end-to-end ileo-colic anastomosis can be performed.

(*b*) When the obstructing lesion lies in the descending colon or sigmoid, a number of alternative procedures are possible including—

(i)   A transverse colostomy, inserting a Paul's tube into the proximal limb in order to deflate the colon as rapidly as possible.

(ii)   A colostomy immediately proximal to the growth is particularly applicable to growths in the sigmoid; the singular advantage claimed for this manoeuvre is that at the time of the definitive resection the colostomy can be included in the resection and the operative management is, therefore, reduced to a two stage procedure.

(iii)   A Paul-Mickulicz procedure. This operation should be reserved for the treatment of obstructing lesions of the sigmoid colon in which hepatic metastases are already present.

(iv)   Caecostomy. In the series reviewed by the author this operation was found to be associated with a high incidence of complications and was abandoned.

The overall mortality, i.e. immediate deaths following the relief of obstruction is high, approximately a third of all patients dying in the immediate postoperative period.

2   *Peritonitis*

Of the 95 patients in the series reviewed, 22 were already moribund on admission and surgical treatment was withheld. In the remainder the best results were obtained when the growth involved the right colon, probably because in this group the causative lesion could be removed. Perforation of a tumour on the left side was normally treated by proximal colostomy and drainage of the affected area.

The mortality of perforated large bowel growths is naturally high because of the gram-negative septicaemia that ensues. In addition, it is now considered that the anaerobic bacteriodes group play a considerable part in contributing to the overall morbidity and mortality of this condition. However, the use of the newer, broad-spectrum antibiotics, together with metranidazole, can in the future be expected to produce a decrease in mortality from the levels of the past which, in the immediate postoperative period, were as high as 70 per cent.

2.7 THE TREATMENT OF MALIGNANT DISEASE BY CYTOTOXIC AGENTS

The benefits that have resulted from the development and introduction of chemotherapeutic antitumour agents have been somewhat limited. However, their introduction has particularly influenced the prognosis of the following tumours—

(*a*)   the lymphomas of the Hodgkin and non-Hodgkin's type;
(*b*)   the leukaemias, in particular acute lymphatic leukaemia;
(*c*)   choriocarcinoma;
(*d*)   certain paediatric tumours including Ewing's sarcoma, Wilm's tumour, glioblastoma multiforme, and Burkitt's tumour.

These, however, account for less than 10 per cent of all malignancies, the other 90 per cent, solid carcinomas and sarcomas, respond poorly if at all. However, it should be remembered that in the latter, cytotoxic agents, if administered at all, are given when all other forms of therapy have failed and in conditions in which studies of cellular kinetics have shown they are at their greatest disadvantage because—

(1)   a large proportion of cells are in the resting (Go phase);
(2)   extensive avascular areas are present which cannot be penetrated by the agent but which are still capable of harbouring viable cells.

NOXIOUS EFFECTS OF CYTOTOXIC AGENTS AND THEIR TREATMENT

1   Haemopoietic effects

Any cytotoxic drug alone or in combination, if given in excess will inevitably cause haemopoietic damage. For this reason a full blood count should be performed on all patients before a drug is administered, and at frequent intervals during treatment. The critical lower values for the various cellular elements in the blood vary somewhat, but in general a white count below 3×10^9/litre and a platelet count below 100×10^9/litre should be viewed with caution. Severe depression of either of these elements can now be treated by white cell or platelet transfusion respectively. Normal blood transfusion is of no value in a thrombocytopenic patient because rapid platelet deterioration occurs in stored blood.

(*a*)   *Platelet transfusion*

A platelet transfusion may be indicated if there is severe uncontrollable haemorrhage during or following a course of chemotherapy. A platelet transfusion is prepared from blood taken from a donor by venesection.

This is then centrifuged to separate the platelets from the other blood components, platelet-phoresis. By this means a platelet rich plasma containing as many as 1.25×10^{11} platelets/500 ml can be obtained. Even further concentration can be achieved by using an even more refined technique so that the transfusion of 500 ml of platelet rich plasma will produce an increase in the circulating platelet count to about $12 \times 10^9/$ m^2 of body surface. The best results from platelet transfusion are obtained when the platelet rich plasma is used within 48 hours. This is because platelets rapidly degenerate even at low temperatures. However, since the life of a transfused platelet is reduced to as little as 2 to 3 days compared with a normal of ten days, repeated transfusions may be necessary. Unfortunately, repeated transfusions can lead to the development of platelet antibodies and platelet transfusion should, therefore, be regarded as a short-term measure only.

(b)   Granulocyte transfusion

The dangers of profound leucopenia are those of infection. Granulocyte transfusions can be used to correct a temporary depletion of the white cells. There are, however, certain difficulties associated with the harvesting of white cells, which have almost the same specific gravity as red cells. The life span of the transfused granulocyte furthermore is short.

An alternative approach to this problem is to isolate the affected patient completely in either a specially designed sterile room or plastic tent and administer antibiotics to sterilise the bowel. Although such methods have been shown to be effective, cost prohibits their general use.

2   Hepatotoxic and nephrotoxic effects

Many chemotherapeutic agents are degraded by the hepatocyte or excreted unchanged by the kidney. Impaired function of either organ may, therefore, lead to higher concentration of the drugs than is normally expected. The result may be myelosuppression followed by uncontrollable bleeding or severe bacterial and fungal infections. Liver function tests and simple tests of renal function should, therefore, always be performed prior to beginning therapy.

3   Gastrointestinal effects

Anorexia, nausea, and vomiting are all significant accompaniments of cytotoxic therapy. These are due to a number of factors which include—

(a)   the psychological effects of cancer therapy.
(b)   the action of these drugs on the brain stem.
(c)   their action on the gastrointestinal tract itself.

Anti-emetics such as metaclopromide (100 mg tds) or in severe cases chlorpromazine (25 mg tds) may help to control these symptoms.

4   Alopecia

No method has yet been found of preventing the development of alopecia. For a short time the use of a scalp tourniquet was popular but it proved generally ineffective. When used it was applied around the forehead and inflated to a pressure of 20 mmHg above the normal systolic blood pressure for a period of up to 30 minutes.

ROUTES OF ADMINISTRATION

The most common methods of administering cytotoxic agents are by the oral or intravenous route but in some instances regional, intracavitary, or the topical application of a drug may be more appropriate.

(a)   Regional chemotherapy

This can be achieved by extracorporeal perfusion or arterial infusion.

Extracorporeal perfusion

This method was specifically designed for treating tumours affecting the limbs. Theoretically it should possess the following advantages—

(i)   because the affected limb is isolated from the general circulation, it should be possible to use very high doses of the selected agent without fear of producing toxic systemic effects;

(ii)   because a pump oxygenator is required, oxygen is supplied at high concentration to the perfused tissue;

(iii)   the limb may be warmed, or vasodilators introduced into the system so that maximum penetration of the tumour-bearing area is achieved by the drug.

Unfortunately, these theoretical advantages are outweighed by the practical disadvantages among which are—

(i)   the requirement for in-patient treatment;

(ii)   the operative risk since major arteries and veins require cannulation and, if perfusing the lower limbs, the aorta must be temporarily occluded;

(iii)   some leakage of the drug always occurs.

Arterial infusion

To use arterial infusion an indwelling arterial catheter or a series of arterial punctures are required. Prior to injecting the agent a radio-opaque dye should be introduced through the cannula in order to ensure that the drug is reaching the desired area.

If methotrexate is the agent of choice in the treatment of a particular tumour the systemic toxic effects can be diminished by administration of large doses of folinic acid within 24 hours.

Arterial perfusion has been used in the treatment of head and neck tumours, secondary liver cancer, malignant melanoma and carcinoma of pancreas, but in general terms the associated complications combined with the increasingly more successful results obtained by intermittent combination therapy have led to the gradual abandonment of this method.

(*b*) **Intracavitary therapy**

Intracavitary therapy has been used to greatest benefit in the treatment of proven malignant effusions of the chest or abdomen.

In every case the drug, usually thiotepa (60 mg) or nitrogen mustard (2 to 10 mg) is inserted into the cavity before the 'tap' is dry so that the agent can spread across the intracavitary lining. Failures are commonplace, particularly in ascitic patients.

Topical therapy

(*a*) *Skin cancer.* Topical cytotoxic therapy is only satisfactory for the treatment of superficial lesions such as Bowen's disease, superficial basal cell carcinomas and erythroplasia of the glans penis. The most commonly used agent is 5 per cent fluoruracil cream, applied twice daily for between two and four weeks.

(*b*) Recently, it has been suggested that suitably diluted cytotoxic agents should be used during the performance of low bowel resections for carcinoma of the colon in order to prevent the local implantation of viable cancer cells which may be shed during the manipulation of the tumour during its mobilisation and subsequent excision.

TREATMENT OF SPECIFIC TUMOURS

1   **The lymphomas**

Indications for the use of cytotoxic agents and the drug schedules used have already been discussed, *see Tutorial Surgery 1,* p.102-104. However, there remain certain other tumours of the haemopoietic system in which cytotoxic agents have been used to considerable advantage; these include—

(a) Chronic lymphatic or myeloid leukaemia

Both these diseases may present to the surgeon with splenomegaly, cause unknown. Both may be treated with cytotoxic agents, although the effects of such treatment are usually more favourable in myeloid leukaemia in which condition the mean survival time following diagnosis is less than two years in the untreated disease. Formerly, chronic myeloid leukaemia was treated by splenic irradiation, which not only reduced splenic size but also induced a remission that was accompanied by a fall in the peripheral white count and correction of the anaemia. However, carefully conducted trials have shown that alkylating agents such as busulphan are somewhat superior to irradiation. Busulphan 2 to 6 mg orally is administered daily until the white count falls to 2×10^9/litre, administration is then stopped. For a few weeks, however, the white count usually continues to fall. Once it has reached 1×10^9/litre a small maintenance dose is required. Unfortunately, chronic myeloid leukaemia usually terminates by transformation into an acute leukaemia.

(b) Polycythaemia rubra vera

This condition is commonly symptomless and may be recognised only because of the rubicund complexion of an individual who is presenting with some unrelated complaint. Alternatively, the patient may present with an apparent vascular problem, complaining of excessive cyanosis of the hands in cold weather, or peripheral venous thromboses apparently occurring without cause. In approximately two-thirds of patients the spleen is palpable.

The diagnosis is confirmed by haematological examination. The chief finding is an increase in the number of circulating red cells when the count commonly exceeds 7×10^{12}/litre. One method of treatment of this condition is by the injection of 5 to 7 milli Curies of the isotope ^{32}P which is selectively concentrated in the bone marrow. Following such an injection the red cell count begins to fall within 6 to 8 weeks and the remission may last for some two years. One objection to this form of treatment is that in some patients the disease terminates in leukaemic transformation, and for this reason cytotoxic agents have been used as an alternative although the total supervision of the patient becomes more difficult because of the need to monitor both the blood count and the dose.

Untreated, approximately 50 per cent of patients die within 18 months whereas with appropriate treatment the 50 per cent survival time is extended to more than ten years.

2 Choriocarcinoma

This is a malignant tumour of the placenta. It may be preceded by a hydatidiform mole, the frequency of which is 1 in 2 000 pregnancies, or arise de novo as a true carcinoma of the chorion, which it does in approximately 1 in 40 000 pregnancies.

Prior to cytotoxic therapy this condition was treated by hysterectomy, if this was possible, followed by irradiation which produced a cure in 40 per cent of patients so long as there were no metastases. Survival in the presence of metastases was negligible.

The cytotoxic agent most widely used is methotrexate, dose 25 mg, orally or intravenously administered daily for 7 days with repeated courses at minimal intervals of one week. Other drugs of value in this condition include actinomycin D, 6-mercaptopurine and the vinca alkaloids. The response to treatment can be monitored by observing the changing secretion of human chorionic gonadotrophin (HCG) which remains present in measurable quantities in the circulation in the presence of clinically undetectable tumour deposits. The presence of circulating HCG indicates that treatment should be continued and this is normally done for several weeks after the final disappearance of the hormone from the circulation.

3 Embryonal tumours

Wilms's tumour

This tumour of the kidney, the nephroblastoma, has a peak incidence between 18 and 24 months and is the fourth most frequent solid malignancy of childhood.

Presentation. (1) A common mode of presentation is as an incidently detected mass often first noted by the mother when dressing her child.

(2) Haematuria, the commonest symptom of an adult renal neoplasm occurs only in about 20 to 30 per cent of cases.

(3) Rare manifestations include:
    (*a*) malignant hypertension due to the production of renin,
    (*b*) polycythaemia due to production of erythropoietin,
    (*c*) pseudo hermaphroditism.

Approximately 4 per cent of Wilms's tumours are bilateral, and pulmonary metastases are already present in about a third of all children when the presence of the tumour is first recognised.

Pathology. Heterologous elements such as smooth or striated muscle are present in about 20 to 30 per cent of all cases. The histological elements and the degree of tumour differentiation are, however, of little prognostic significance as compared to the importance of staging since, if the tumour is limited to kidney, 80 per cent of children survive.

Treatment. Prior to the use of chemotherapy the overall survival rate when surgical excision was combined with radiotherapy, was of the order of 40 per cent. The latter, usually given postoperatively, could also be administered preoperatively in order to reduce a tumour to more surgically manageable proportions.

Chemotherapy. The drug first found to be of value in the treatment of Wilms's tumour was actinomycin-D but the tumour may also respond to the vinca alkaloids and cyclophosphamide. The finding that at least 50 per cent of children were already suffering from occult metastases at the time of their initial presentation led to the suggestion that this drug should be given to all children regardless of the operative findings. Such treatment produced an improvement in the 4-year survival figures to over 60 per cent.

Initially given at the time of surgery, chemotherapy is now commonly administered in courses of treatment at 6 weeks, 12 weeks, and then, thereafter, at 3-monthly intervals until a total of six courses has been given over 15 months. The prognosis is usually good should the child survive to an age equal to twice its years at detection plus the nine months gestation period, 'Colin's rule.'

Medulloblastoma

This is one of the most common tumours of childhood, the yearly mortality being approximately equal to that of all bone sarcomas, Wilms's tumour, and lymphocytic lymphoma put together.

Presentation. The mean age of presentation is between 6 and 8 years of age although the first manifestations may occur from the neonatal period onwards. The common symptoms and signs arise from the increasing intracranial pressure.

Pathology. This tumour arises from the external layer of Obersteiner and most commonly involves the roof of the fourth ventricle; it is composed of dense sheets of small basophilic cells with occasional rosette formation. A particular characteristic is that it may spread to involve the whole of the central nervous system.

Treatment. Normally, treatment following diagnosis is by radiotherapy but such tumours have been shown to be sensitive to methotrexate, the vinca alkaloids, and the nitrosoureas. The last-named possess the theoretical advantage of lipid solubility, a property that allows them to cross the blood brain barrier.

Rhadomyosarcoma

This tumour accounts for only about 10 per cent of solid tumours in children.

Pathology. Although localised in striated muscle, these tumours probably arise from primitive mesenchymal tissues. They are often associated with a non-neoplastic proliferation of the surface epithelium with the result that they have a polypoid appearance, hence the name sarcoma botryoides for those tumours involving the vagina of the female child. Other common sites in which this rare tumour originates are the orbit and, in older children, any skeletal muscle. The overall survival rate is extremely low. Histologically these tumours consist of spindle-cell or pleomorphic sarcoma-like cells in a myxomatous stroma.

Treatment. These tumours have been shown to be sensitive to the vinca alkaloids, actinomycin D and some of the alkylating agents. At the present time, various systems of combination chemotherapy of up to two years duration, with doxorubicin, are being used with increasing lengths of survival in about 60 per cent of children so treated.

4   Lymphocytic lymphoma (Burkitt's tumour)

Clinical features. First described by Burkitt, in 1958, in African children between 2 and 14 years of age, this tumour has several distinctive features.
1   50 per cent affect the jaws;
2   in the remainder almost any site in the body may be affected;
3   it is commonest in low-lying, moist tropical areas, and although first described in Africa it is also found in New Guinea and Columbia.

Pathology. Histologically it resembles other diffuse lymphocytic lymphomata in that there are numerous palely staining histiocytes among the lymphocytic cells producing a 'starry-sky' appearance.

Aetiology. Burkitt's tumour is associated with a herpes virus known as the EB virus after Epstein and Barr who first isolated it in 1964. This virus has been cultured from the neoplastic cells and all patients have a high titre of antibodies to the virus. However, the same virus has been established as the cause of infectious mononucleosis with a positive Paul-Bunnell reaction, and it may, therefore, be merely a passenger, rather than the cause of the condition.

Staging. The staging system used for the clinical classification of the extent of the disease closely resembles that used for Hodgkin's disease and is as follows—

Stage I   Disease limited to one anatomical area.
Stage II   (a) disease limited to two contiguous areas;
               (b) disease occurring in two or more non-adjacent areas but
               on the same side of the diaphragm;
Stage III   (a) disease involving structures on both sides of the dia-
               phragm;
               (b) generalised bone marrow involvement.
Stage IV   Central nervous system involvement.

Treatment. The most valuable and successful drugs in the treatment of
Burkitt's lymphoma are the alkylating agents, especially cyclophosphamide, although many other drugs exert a beneficial influence on the
disease. In Stages 1 and 2 it has been reported that a single injection of
cyclophosphamide, 40 mg/kg will produce a remission but in the later
stages of the disease repeated courses are required. Failure to respond, or
subsequent relapse after treatment, demand the use of repeated courses
using combination therapy. Long-term relapse following apparently
successful therapy is not unknown but after a two-year disease-free interval the relapse rate falls rapidly.

Solid tumours of the adult

In general, the beneficial effects of cytotoxic therapy in the treatment of
solid tumours of the adult have been disappointing, although in some
tumours such as carcinoma of the breast aggressive combination therapy
may cause a remission for a limited period of time in about half the
patients. In contrast, bronchial carcinoma, which is the commonest cause
of death from cancer in the UK at the present time, appears to be relatively refractory to chemotherapeutic agents and the value of such
treatment is open to debate.

Carcinoma of breast

Adjuvant therapy. So far as carcinoma of the breast is concerned the 'great
debate' revolves around the use of adjuvant therapy in premenopausal
patients presenting with Stage I and Stage II disease. In Stage I, using
conventional therapy, a 5 year survival of approximately 80 per cent can
be expected, but at 10 years this has fallen to 70 per cent. In Stage II the
comparable figures are approximately 40 per cent survival at 5 years and
30 per cent at 10 years.
    The argument in favour of adjuvant therapy, therefore, appears un-
deniable, since our knowledge of tumour kinetics suggests that the smaller
the initial tumour mass the greater the ultimate chance of achieving a cure.

In advanced disease. In advanced breast cancer, intermittent combination
chemotherapy produces the most satisfactory results. One advantage such

treatment possesses over the various hormonal preparations is its comparatively rapid action so that in a responsive tumour some benefit may be seen in as little as two to three weeks. Treatment can be administered as an outpatient and, typical of the many combinations that have been suggested is the following regime—

Day 1   Start oral cyclophosphamide, 50 mg twice daily. Administer 500 mg 5-fluorouracil, 25 mg methotrexate and 5 mg vinblastine sequentially via an intravenous drip of 300 ml of sodium chloride.

Day 8   Repeat the infusion.

Day 15   Cease cyclophosphamide and repeat infusion.

Leave four weeks without treatment and then repeat the cycle if the white blood count remains above 3×10^9/litre.

2.8 INDICATIONS FOR LOWER LIMB AMPUTATION, THE SITES OF MAJOR AMPUTATIONS, AND COMMON COMPLICATIONS

Indications

In the absence of war with its associated trauma, the common indications for amputations in the lower limb are obliterative arterial disease, tumours, trauma, chronic infection, irremediable paralysis, cosmetic deformity, and congenital deformities. Approximately 70 per cent of all amputations performed in the developed countries are for obliterative arterial disease, usually caused by atherosclerosis, less commonly by Buerger's disease, and least commonly by diabetes in the absence of large vessel disease.

Sites of lower limb amputations

The sites at which lower limb amputations may be performed are hindquarter, hip disarticulation, above knee, transcondylar, through knee, below knee, Symes's amputation, and distal amputations either of a single toe, or the toe together with the corresponding metatarsal.

When considering the possible site of an amputation, two opposing philosophies are at work. Occasionally, the site is obligatory, particularly when it concerns treatment of a malignant tumour. Otherwise the site of amputation is governed by two factors—

(a)   the desire of the surgeon to achieve a low mortality together with primary healing of the wound;

(b)   the patient's aspiration to become mobile following amputation.

As a general rule the more distal the amputation the more easily does the patient attain mobility. However, even an apparently simple amputation such as excision of the first toe and metatarsal may be followed by enormous difficulties due to pain and alterations in the dynamics of the metatarsal arch.

AMPUTATION IN PERIPHERAL VASCULAR DISEASE

In this condition approximately 14 per cent of symptomatic sufferers finally come to amputation, usually due to the development of intolerable rest pain or gangrene.

Mortality

Although different series report widely differing mortality rates for various amputations there is little doubt that above-knee amputations are followed by a higher mortality than below-knee, and that the rehabilitation of above-knee amputees is much more difficult than that of below-knee. In one recently reported series the mortality of above-knee amputations was 28 per cent as compared to 10 per cent for below-knee, and the ability to walk following unilateral amputation was 46 per cent for above-knee amputees as compared to 76 per cent for below-knee.

Primary healing

So far as primary healing is concerned, above-knee amputation has found most favour in atherosclerotic gangrene because the rate of primary healing of the stump is high, 75 to 85 per cent, delayed healing occurring in the remainder. However, below-knee amputation is gaining in popularity because it has been shown that if a long posterior skin flap is fashioned, without detaching it from the underlying muscles, a high primary healing rate can be achieved. It has been suggested that as many as 60 per cent of patients suffering from atherosclerotic gangrene could undergo a below-knee amputation.

If a below-knee amputation is planned, the following points must be considered—

1 the femoral pulse should be palpable;
2 there should be no flexion deformity at the knee joint;
3 the skin and subcutaneous tissues should not be affected by the ischaemic lesion at the site of the skin flap construction;
4 there should be good bleeding at the site of amputation.

TECHNIQUE OF ABOVE-KNEE AND BELOW-KNEE AMPUTATIONS

Both above and below-knee elective amputations are usually performed by a myoplastic technique originally promoted by Dederich and Mondry.

The site of election for above-knee amputations is 10 to 12 in (25 to 30 cm) below the greater trochanter, and in an adult the stump must terminate 10 to 12½ cm above the axis of the knee joint in order to provide room for a movable prosthetic device. Below the knee the site of election is 5½ in (14 cm) below the tibial plateau, and this amputation is rarely effective if the stump is less than 9 cm long.

In an above-knee amputation the adductors are stitched to the abductors over the bone end, following which the flexors and extensors are sutured together. The advantage of this technique is better adherence of the stump to the socket, and the prominent bone end is eliminated.

When the same technique is applied to a below-knee amputation a transverse skin incision is made on the anterior surface of the limb 11.5 cm below the knee joint, extending for one-third of the circumference of the leg. The incision is then carried distally along the axis of the limb on each side for a distance of 15 cm. The two limbs of this incision are then joined to make a long posterior flap. The tibia is divided 14 cm below the knee joint and the fibula 2.5 cm proximal to this. The soleus and gastrocnemius are dissected from the tibia, after which the bulk of the muscle is reduced by an oblique slice, using a Syme's amputation knife cutting through the muscle in a downwards and backwards direction.

In both amputations the nerves are divided proximal to other tissues in an attempt to prevent neuromas developing.

Particularly with above-knee amputation, preoperative training, if possible, greatly shortens the period required for rehabilitation. In the early postoperative period both stumps should be carefully bandaged to ensure that they are moulded into a conical shape, and postoperative exercises should be performed in order to prevent the development of contractures and deformity.

Alternative procedures

From time to time, two other major amputations have been strongly advocated. The Stokes-Gritti amputation performed through the level of the femoral condyles. In the initial description of this amputation the patella was preserved after shaving the articular cartilage from the posterior surface, following which the raw surfaces of the two bones were opposed. This step in the operation is now considered unnecessary and has been abandoned because it requires considerable time for union to occur between the femur and the patella, the rate of non-union is high and, lastly, the patella often tends to slip off the end of the femur, producing an irregular and tender stump difficult to fit with a prosthesis.

The second alternative major amputation is the through-knee. The advantages claimed for this amputation are that it gives an end weight-

111

bearing stump, that it is relatively bloodless, and that the resulting limb is powerful because the majority of muscles are left intact.

The disadvantages of a through-knee amputation are—

(*a*) that the stump is bulbous, hence difficult to fit with a convenient and cosmetic prosthesis;

(*b*) the excessive length prohibits the use of a swing phase controlled prosthetic knee mechanism;

(*c*) it requires as much skin for coverage as the short below-knee stump which provides a better functional result.

Neither of these operations has gained general acceptance.

DISTAL AMPUTATION

In the foot, 'ray' amputations removing a gangrenous toe, together with the appropriate metatarsal, are often successful in dealing with diabetic gangrene so long as the large blood vessels are patent. If there is considerable soft tissue infection the wound can always be left open and a delayed primary or secondary suture performed.

COMPLICATIONS OF AMPUTATION

Amputations are associated with a great many complications.

1   *Conditions of the skin*

(*a*) delayed healing due to ischaemia;

(*b*) chronic ulceration, which may be due to underlying osteomyelitis, adherence of the skin to the underlying bone, or ischaemia of the flaps;

(*c*) staphylococcal infections of the stump;

(*d*) dermatitis, eczema, and intertrigo;

(*e*) sinus formation due either to chronic osteomyelitis or the use of non-absorbable sutures.

2   *Conditions of the bone*

(*a*) cross union between two bones. This is of no importance in the lower limb but should it happen in the forearm, fusion of the radius and ulna leads to loss of function;

(*b*) spur formation, which causes pain and the formation of adventitous bursae;

(*c*) in a growing child the bone end may perforate the skin;

112

(*d*)   osteomyelitis with sequestrum formation may produce a sinus or chronic ulceration.

3   Conditions of muscles

Contractures, leading to deformity and inability to wear prosthesis. In above-knee amputations the commonest deformity of the stump is fixed flexion and abduction, because the adductors and the hamstring muscles have been divided. In below-knee amputations a fixed flexion deformity can also develop.

4   Idiopathic conditions

(*a*)   phantom limb;
(*b*)   painful phantom, the pain of which may possibly be alleviated by percussion;
(*c*)   a painful neuroma;
(*d*)   causalgia (for treatment *see* section on Intractable Pain.)

2.9   HAEMOSTATIC DEFECTS OF SPECIAL INTEREST TO THE SURGEON

1   Haemophilia

Inheritance

Prior to 1911, the term haemophilia was used to describe any inherent haemorrhagic condition. The work of Bullock and Fildes, however, separated this specific entity from all other conditions associated with an abnormal bleeding tendency, and in 1936 Patek and Taylor demonstrated that the essential factor missing from the blood was associated with neither platelets nor fibrinogen.

The condition is normally inherited as a sex-linked recessive characteristic, the male exhibiting the disease and the female acting as a carrier and transmitting the disease to the next generation. The female heterozygote is usually unaffected because she is protected by the normal allele on her second X chromosome. In the male, however, the heterozygote is affected since the Y does not carry the allele. The disease may occur in the female, but only following the mating of an affected male with a female carrier. Approximately one-third of all cases occur in the absence of a family history suggesting that spontaneous mutation may occur.

Pathology

The underlying pathological feature of haemophilia is a deficiency of the procoagulant activity of Factor VIII, which can be as low as 1 to 2 per cent of normal. A protein recognised immunologically as 'Factor VIII related antigen' is always present but without coagulant activity. A similar deficiency in Factor IX causes the much rarer Christmas disease, sometimes called Haemophilia B to distinguish it from the classical haemophilia, often referred to as Haemophilia A. The latter is ten times commoner than the former but it is still a rare condition affecting only about 6 of 100,000 of the population, hence about 3000 cases exist in the United Kingdom.

A third variant is von Willebrand's disease, a condition in which both sexes are equally affected and in which the bleeding time is prolonged because of a platelet defect accompanied by abnormal platelet adhesion and aggregation plus a Factor VIII deficiency.

Measurement of severity of haemophilia

The clinical severity of haemophilia is determined by the reduced plasma factor .VIII activity. If many members of the family are involved, the severity of the defect appears to be the same in all those affected.

The unit of measurement used to assess the disease is the international unit of factor VIII; one international unit is based on the activity of 1 ml of average fresh normal plasma, also described as having 100 per cent activity. In a normal individual, factor VIII activity varies between 60 to 75 per cent of the mean. Individuals with levels between 26 and 40 per cent are, in practice, unlikely to bleed unless subjected to major surgery or trauma; 6 to 25 per cent indicates mild haemophilia with a tendency to bleed only if injured. If, however, the level reaches between 1 and 5 per cent, bleeding will follow minor trauma and haemarthroses are likely; below this level the disease is particularly severe and spontaneous bleeding can be expected.

Clinical symptoms

Haemophilia is most commonly diagnosed in early childhood when either excessive bruising or persistent bleeding after minor trauma or surgery may be noticed. In severe cases, see below, the presenting symptom may be the development of painful deep haematomata. Occurring in the neck, such haematomata may lead to asphyxia, and in the soft tissues in general the vascular or nervous supply to an area may be compromised by the increasing tension developing in a compartment surrounded by deep fascia. Severe bleeding followed eventually by fibrosis may lead to contractures and subsequent deformity. Typical would be an equinus deformity of the foot following bleeding into the posterior compartment of the leg, or a

Volkmann's contracture of the forearm and hand if bleeding occurs in the upper limb.

Bleeding into the joints themselves is also a characteristic feature of severe haemophilia. Severe pain may occur due to stretching of the joint capsule, and a large haemarthrosis will be extremely painful, tender to touch or pressure, and swollen and warm so that in the absence of any previous history the condition must be distinguished from a septic arthritis. Blood mixed with synovial fluids acts as an irritant to the synovial membrane with the result that, eventually, when large quantities of haemosiderin have been deposited in the subsynovial tissues, a reactive granulation tissue develops and forms a pannus which gradually extends over and absorbs the articular cartilage. At the same time the deposition of iron in the cartilage itself leads to degeneration, the cartilage becoming soft and yellowish and unable to withstand stress. This results in breakdown and irregularity of the cartilage, which develops a map-like appearance and the subchondral cortex tends to thin out and form cysts. The hyperaemia in the growth period causes enlargement of the epiphyses of the affected joints, commonly in an asymmetrical fashion, so that gross deformities develop. The overall rate of growth may be either increased or retarded. In addition to actual haemarthroses, subperiosteal haemorrhages may lead to pseudo-tumours. Ill-advised aspiration or biopsy of either joint or haematoma may lead to infection. The joints most commonly affected are the knees, ankles, elbows, and hips in that order, and while the acute stage may last for days or weeks the chronic synovitis that follows the haemarthrosis may persist for weeks or months.

When considering the alleviation of pain in the haemophiliac it must be remembered that many of the common analgesics and anti-inflammatory drugs inhibit platelet aggregation and prolong bleeding time, hence the use of aspirin to prevent deep venous thrombosis. Thus, aspirin, indomethecin and phenylbutazone should be avoided and the relief of pain sought in pentazocine, or in one of the narcotic group of drugs if the pain is very severe.

Retroperitoneal bleeding is also possible and may follow mild abdominal trauma or even strenuous exercise. The ability of the retroperitoneal space to hold large quantities of blood may result in the development of haemorrhagic shock and the appearance of Cullen's or Grey-Turner's signs both of which are more commonly associated with acute haemorrhagic pancreatitis or a ruptured abdominal aortic aneurysm.

Diagnosis

The diagnosis of haemophilia should always be suspected in a patient with a bleeding tendency and a classical family history in whom a normal platelet count is found, along with a normal bleeding and prothrombin time. However, further investigation shows that the Kaolin Cephalin time is prolonged and accompanied by reduced prothrombin and lower levels of Factor VIII and IX, the levels of the latter being measured by direct assay.

Treatment

The indications for surgical intervention in the haemophiliac are precisely the same as in a normal individual except for those patients in whom antibodies to Factor VIII have developed due to previous treatment. Basically, should the haemophiliac suffer a major bleed or require surgery then the defective level of AHG should be made good by replacement therapy so that the level exceeds the 30 per cent level. It was first demonstrated in 1955 that the condition could be controlled by the use of fresh blood or plasma, 1000 ml of the latter raising the AHG from 0 to 15 per cent. However, following the administration of a given dose of Factor VIII, approximately half of the initial post-transfusion activity disappears from the plasma within four hours. This disappearance is thought to be due for the most part to diffusion from the intravascular space. The period of equilibration extends for about eight hours, after which only about 25 per cent of the initial level remains. Thereafter the slope is less steep, but after 24 hours only about 10 per cent of the administered activity remains.

One unit of Factor VIII activity is defined as that amount present in 1 ml of fresh normal plasma, and is expressed as a percentage in that 100 IU/100 ml = 100 per cent, although the range of normal varies from 40 per cent to 180 per cent. Thus, assuming that the initial concentration of AHG was zero, to achieve a level of 30 per cent of normal, using fresh plasma, a volume of plasma equal to 30 per cent of the estimated plasma volume would be needed and, because of the natural loss already described, at least one half of the initial volume would need to be administered every twelve hours. Such volumes are excessive, and the use of fresh plasma or fresh frozen plasma has now been replaced by the use of cryoprecipitate or AHG concentrate. Cryoprecipitation was developed from observing that a cold precipitate of plasma was rich in AHG. Fresh plasma is snap frozen and then thawed at 4°C, when a stringy precipitate, the cryoprecipitate is left in the plasma. This contains approximately 50 per cent of the AHG of the original material but still contains very variable amounts of AHG.

The supernatant plasma is removed and the cryoprecipitate is then frozen. AHG concentrate in a lyophilised state is the material of choice administered by most haemophilia authorities to haemophiliac patients bleeding or requiring major surgery. It has the advantage over cryoprecipitate in that the amount of AHG administered is known exactly, as the batches of AHG concentrate have been assayed for Factor VIII content. These materials come in vials containing about 250 units of Factor VIII and are stable for many months at 4°C. For use, the material is dissolved in 10 to 20 ml of sterile water, enabling effective haemostatic doses to be injected in a small volume.

The formula for the amount of Factor VIII to be administered as recommended by Biggs is as follows:

$$\text{Total units of Factor VIII required} = \frac{\text{Wt in kg} \times \text{the desired Factor VIII rise (as per cent)}}{\text{k } 1.5}$$

The dose required and the frequency with which it should be given are determined by the type of operation, the weight of the patient and by the fact that the half-life of Factor VIII is about 12 hours. In a surgical setting, the initial level of Factor VIII should first be assayed so that adequacy of the calculated dose can be determined and throughout the course of treatment the assay should be repeated at intervals. The aim of treatment, particularly if the patient is to undergo major surgery, is to obtain an initial plasma level above 0.8 IU/ml (80 per cent of normal) and then maintain the level above 40 per cent for some seven to ten days by repeated administration of AHG at 12 hourly intervals.

Complications of therapy

1 Serum hepatitis;
2 Development of inhibitors that neutralise AHG activity.
Their presence should be suspected when an apparently adequate dose of Factor VIII raises the plasma level only slightly, transiently, or not at all. Various workers have found the incidence of inhibitors to be between 5 to 21 per cent. Their development makes treatment of the individual exceedingly complicated, if not impossible.

Bovine and porcine preparations have also been used, but these also stimulate antibody formation in the majority of patients. Should, however, antibodies to human AHG be present in a life-threatening situation animal preparations can be used. Recent reports suggest that activated Factor IX concentrates are of considerable value when high concentrations of inhibitor prevent the use of AHG. The basis of such therapy is that these concentrates contain certain activated factors which may bypass the point of action of Factor VIII in the haemostatic process and thus make the presence of antibody of no consequence.

Allergic reactions

These also are relatively rare. The reaction usually occurs during or within 1 to 2 hours. The symptoms may consist of headaches, backache, urticaria, rigor, fever and tightness in the chest, and, rarely, pulmonary oedema. Minor reactions may be treated by antihistamines, and major reactions accompanied by bronchospasm with subcutaneous adrenaline and intravenous hydrocortisone.

2   Factor IX deficiency: Christmas disease, Haemophilia B

Christmas disease is clinically indistinguishable from Factor VIII deficiency and was recognised only in 1952. It is, however, a much less common condition than Factor VIII deficiency and affects only approximately 1 per 1,000,000 of the population. Like Haemophilia A, Christmas disease is also inherited as a sex-linked recessive characteristic; it mimics haemophilia A so closely that it can be differentiated only by a direct assay of Factor IX.

Recently, Factor IX concentrates have become available in most haemophiliac centres for clinical use.

3 Von Willebrand's disease

This condition, first described by von Willebrand in the inhabitants of the Aland Islands in the Baltic Sea, has aroused considerable interest.

The disease is inherited as an autosomal dominant trait and, therefore, appears in consecutive generations affecting both males and females equally.

Clinical presentation and pathology

The condition is characterised by bleeding from mucous membranes, haemarthroses, and postoperative haemorrhage.

The three abnormal haematological features are a prolonged bleeding time, reduced platelet adhesiveness, and a diminished Factor VIII activity which, although always present, is never as great as in classic haemophilia. Also, whereas in the latter the AHG level, whatever its concentration, tends to remain constant, in patients with von Willebrand's disease it seems to vary appreciably from time to time. Similarly, although a prolonged bleeding time is nearly always present it, too, varies considerably.

Aetiology and treatment

von Willebrand's disease is due to a deficiency of 'Factor VIII related antigen'. In this disease, once this factor is transfused into a patient he or she can then produce Factor VIII procoagulant activity. Within 4 to 6 hours posttransfusion, the activity of Factor VIII can rise by a factor of 5 to 8 and this synthesis may continue for a period of 25 hours. This response can be obtained even following the transfusion of haemophiliac plasma because the haemophiliac has the 'Factor VIII related antigen'. In summary, therefore, haemophilia A has a reduced procoagulant activity but the Factor VIII related antigen is normal, whereas in von Willebrand's disease the procoagulant activity is normal but the 'Factor VIII antigen' is reduced.

4 Bleeding associated with liver disease

Since the liver is the site of all protein production, with the exception of the immunoglobulins, it is hardly surprising that liver disease will cause disturbances in haemostasis. Furthermore, the liver normally removes active coagulation factors and, therefore, helps to maintain normal haemostatic balance.

(*a*) To the general surgeon, the most common disturbance causing difficulty is the presence of obstructive jaundice. Absence of bile salts from the lumen of the small intestine leads to failure of absorption of the fat soluble vitamin K, with the result that the synthesis of vitamin K dependent factors is blocked. The low plasma levels of these factors causes a marked prolongation of the prothrombin time which must be corrected prior to operation by the parenteral administration of vitamin K_1 (phytomenadione).

(*b*) In patients suffering from severe liver disease such as hepatic necrosis or severe alcoholic cirrhosis not only the vitamin K dependent factors but also Factor V and the fibrinogen level may be disturbed. Such patients represent a severe haemostatic risk and require not only vitamin K but also fresh blood, fresh frozen plasma, and platelet concentrates.

5   **Difficulties associated with extra corporeal circulation**

Many haemostatic parameters are disturbed by the prolonged use of cardiopulmonary bypass. The aetiology of the haemostatic defect is usually multifactorial and consists of the inadequate neutralisation of heparin, thrombocytopenia and the development of clotting factor deficiencies chiefly involving Factors II, V and VIII.

6   **Disseminated intravascular coagulation** (Defibrination syndrome)

This condition is due to widespread activation of the coagulation factors of the blood. When acute there is usually a sudden onset of purpura, or loss of blood from the gastrointestinal, urinary, or genital tracts. In the chronic condition thrombotic manifestations may predominate.

This condition is always secondary to some underlying cause, and of greatest importance to the surgeon is its occurrence in—
(*a*)   shock, especially Bacteraemic shock;
(*b*)   burns;
(*c*)   disseminated malignancy;
(*d*)   following cardiac arrest and resuscitation.

Pathogenesis

The condition is the result of clot-promoting substances entering the circulation, the products of tissue trauma, aminiotic fluid embolism, snake venom, endotoxins, or antigen-antibody complexes arising from a variety of cells which then release procoagulant materials into the blood stream.

The release of these factors into the circulation results in the generation of thrombin. From this moment onwards a complex series of reactions occur in the blood with the result that not only is there widespread coagulation but also widespread bleeding.

Treatment

(*a*) removal or treatment of the causal agent if possible;
(*b*) if persistent bleeding occurs, administer whole fresh blood;
(*c*) replace the lost clotting factors by fresh frozen plasma;
(*d*) the possible administration of heparin to arrest further intravascular coagulation.

2.10 THE 'SURGICAL' PARASITES

1   HYDATID DISEASE

Geographical distribution

The highest incidence of this disease occurs in those geographical areas that are most densely populated by the intermediate host of the parasite, the sheep. This disease, therefore, is most commonly found in Australia, New Zealand and Southern Africa. In Britain, the disease is somewhat commoner in Wales than elsewhere. The cause of hydatid disease is a tapeworm.

Causal Agents

Hydatid disease is caused by the tapeworms, *Echinococcus granulosus* and *E. multilocularis*. The latter, which is much less common, is found only in the colder climatic conditions of Alaska and Russia and neither can infect man in any area unless personal hygiene is substandard.

Life cycle (Fig. 2.10)

Man is infected by the worm only by accident since the natural cycle is between the dog and the sheep, the latter acting as the intermediate host. This natural cycle stems from the domestic dog eating sheep offal contaminated by hydatid cysts. The scolices within the cysts adhere to the wall of the small intestine and develop into the adult tapeworm which consists of only four segments including the head, on which are two rows of hooklets and four sucking pads. These enable the worm to adhere to

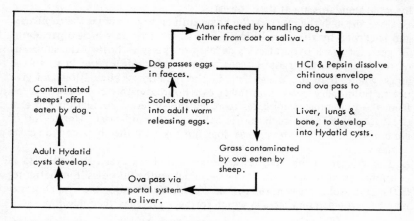

Fig 2.10   Life cycle of **Echinococcus granulosus**

the wall of the bowel. An adult worm is between 3 and 5 mm in length and the gravid terminal segments are shed by the worm (Fig. 2.11). The dog's faeces adhere to its fur and generally contaminate the environment.

The life cycle is normally completed when sheep eat the eggs or gravid segments. Dissolution of the chitinous coat liberates a hexacanth embryo which then burrows into and through the wall of the intestine. In a similar manner the human is infected by eating materials contaminated by the excreta of dogs, an incident most likely to occur in childhood when hygienic standards are at their lowest.

Once through the mucosa, the hexacanth embryo invades the capillaries and is carried by the portal blood, first to the liver in which organ about 70 per cent of all hydatid cysts develop or, passing through the sinusoids of the liver, the embryos proceed via the right side of the heart to the lungs where they are caught up in the pulmonary circulation and give rise to pulmonary cysts. Still fewer ova, approximately 5 per cent, escape from the pulmonary capillaries to reach the systemic circulation and give rise to cysts in areas such as the spleen, brain and bone. Unlike the *E. granulosus*, the *E. multilocularis* does not produce the characteristic cysts of the former.

The danger facing man is that once a hydatid cyst has developed it continues to grow until the lining germinal epithelium dies. Furthermore, if the cyst wall is broken, the germinal epithelium and/or the cyst contents may be carried to new sites in which further cysts may then develop.

Pathology of the cyst (Fig. 2.12)

The cyst developed from the embryo is composed of three layers—

(*a*) The outer adventitial layer or ectocyst derived from host tissues which may eventually calcify.

(*b*) The intermediate or laminated layer.

(*c*) The inner or germinal layer forming the brood capsules from which the scolices are developed.

The brood capsules form from nodes of multiplying cells in the germinal layer which becomes vacuolated and pedunculated. Scolices develop from a thickening of the lining of the brood capsule and eventually indent it. As the brood capsules increase in size so their attachment to the germinal layer becomes progressively thinner until, finally, the capsule bursts, releasing the scolices into the fluid of the cyst. Alternatively, a fertile hydatid daughter cyst may bud off externally and become separated, forming a secondary cyst. A scolex (Fig. 2.13) has suckers, hooklets and a body; ingested by the dog it is able to adhere to the mucosa of the small intestine and develop into an adult tapeworm.

The majority of embryos reaching the liver excite a host reaction which is sufficient to kill them, after which they are removed by phagocytosis. Only a minority survive and, in man, growth of the cystic

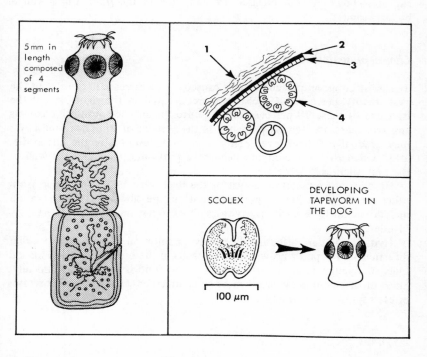

5mm in length composed of 4 segments

1
2
3
4

SCOLEX

DEVELOPING TAPEWORM IN THE DOG

100 µm

Left
Fig 2.11   Adult tapeworm developed in dog's intestine

Top right
Fig 2.12   Hydatid cyst developing in man or sheep
1. Adventitious wall derived from host
2. External laminated layer
3. Internal germinal layer
4. Brood capsule containing scolices

Bottom right
Fig 2.13   Developing tapeworm in intestine of dog

123

larval stage is so slow that an infection acquired in childhood may not be clinically apparent until early adult life by which time the periparasitic tissues have been gradually converted into fibrous tissue. So slow is the growth of the cyst that one year after infection the cyst may be only about 4 cm in diameter.

The fluid contained in a cyst is normally clear and contains a little protein which is secreted by the germinal membrane. After a brood cyst ruptures, however, the released scolices float in the fluid, the so-called hydatid sand.

Clinical presentation

The most common presentation is caused by an increase in the size of the cyst. Eighty per cent of such cysts are situated in the right lobe of the liver and of these 70 per cent project onto the anterior or inferior aspects and are, therefore, readily palpable. In the absence of complications a cyst may gradually enlarge over many years until eventually the larvae die, after which the cyst contents become a putty-like mass and the wall of the cyst calcifies.

On clinical examination a cyst of the liver must be distinguished from other swellings in the upper quadrant of the abdomen. These would include conditions such as hydronephrosis and mucocele of the gall-bladder.

Hydatid disease affecting bones is uncommon. There is a peculiar diverticulated type of growth which results in the production of semisolid buds of hyaline tissue in which little or no fluid is produced. Clinically, bone involvement may result in bone enlargement, paraosseous abscesses or even spontaneous fractures.

Diagnosis

(*a*)   Plain X-rays may reveal hepatomegaly. In some cases calcification of the cyst wall makes the diagnosis obvious. The diaphragm is often grossly distorted and a pleural effusion may be present.

(*b*)   Ultrasonography demonstrates the presence of a 'cystic' space-occupying lesion (*see* p. 150).

(*c*)   *Casoni's Test.* This intradermal test becomes positive because the capsule is semipermeable and allows the protein containing hydatid fluid which is antigenic to leak into the general circulation. The test, therefore, is performed by injecting a little hydatid fluid intradermally into the patient under investigation, the presence of antibodies being revealed by the rapid development of a skin reaction.

(*d*)   *Aspiration.* Aspiration followed by microscopic examination of the contents of the cyst is helpful if scolices or hooklets can be found in the aspirate. This investigation, however, may lead to leakage of hydatid fluid from the cyst and be followed by an anaphylactic reaction.

Treatment

The only possible treatment of hepatic cysts is removal. The liver is exposed, the cyst is partially emptied by aspiration, and the contents are replaced by 10 ml of pure formalin in order to kill any contained scolices, although the daughter cysts remain unaffected. The operation field is then packed with gauze soaked in 10 per cent formalin and the whole of the cyst contents are removed by suction. The liver substance is then divided and the cyst gently removed by dissection in the plane between the hyaline and advential layers.

Cysts in the lung may be treated in the same fashion when they are situated at the periphery. Occasionally, when they are situated in a deep parabronchial position, they undergo natural cure by expectoration.

Complications

(*a*)   *Rupture.* Rupture of a cyst may cause hydatid anaphylaxis accompanied by an erythematous urticarial rash.

(*b*)   *Infection.* Infection may occur in either a dead or a living cyst.

2   SCHISTOSOMIASIS

Causal agents

Three species of schistosome, or bloodfluke, infect man and are responsible for the chronic disease known as schistosomiasis—

(*a*)   *Schistosoma haematobium*, common throughout the African continent and the Middle East and in endemic foci in Egypt, and West and East Africa.

(*b*)   *S. mansoni*, common in South America and Africa.

(*c*)   *S. japonicum*, confined to the Far East.

The schistosome is a blood fluke which lives in the vascular system, *S. haematobium* favouring the venous channels of the lower ureters; *S. mansoni* and *S. japonicum* are associated with the venous tributaries of the gut. In endemic areas such as Egypt the extension of irrigation systems has solved the problem of water shortage but increased the overall danger of infection by the schistosome.

125

SCHISTOSOMA HAEMATOBIUM

Life cycle and pathology (Fig. 2.14)

The intermediate host *S. haematobium* is the fresh water snail, *Bulinus globosus*, which is infected by the free-swimming miracidia liberated from eggs passed in the urine of an infected human. In the snail's liver the miracidia develop into sporocysts in which the fork-tailed cercariae form. These tiny hair-like creatures, about a millimetre in length, leave the snail in thousands, usually during daylight hours. The definitive host, man, is infected by the cercariae penetrating the skin. This usually occurs when the host is wading or bathing in water that contains the cercariae, which have only a lifespan of about 12 hours.

Penetration is marked by an urticarial reaction which lasts from 1 to 2 days. Once through the skin, the cercariae shed their tails and invade the lymphatic system and so eventually gain access to the blood stream. Carried to the liver the cercariae settle in the portal system and there mature into either male or female flukes. This is followed by a secondary migration to the site of election during which a generalised allergic reaction may occur. The *S. haematobium* passes to the venules of the bladder and surrounding pelvic viscera, and in the perivesical venules the female, gripped in the gynaecophoral groove of the male, lays her eggs. The nonoperculate eggs, which possess spines, the position of which reflects the species, penetrate the walls of the venules and pass into the substance of the bladder wall.

At this stage there are two possibilities:

(*a*) the egg may lyse its way through the wall of the bladder and slowly develop into the miracidial stage, ready to hatch once the egg has been passed in the urine; or

(*b*) the egg will be retained in the bladder wall and ultimately die.

Whatever occurs, the eggs always excite a granulomatous reaction in the affected tissues. The typical lesion consists of a focus of epithelioid cells, fibroblasts, and giant cells surrounded by plasma cells and lymphocytes. Should the egg die, fibrosis and calcification occur at the site, the degree depending on the intensity of infection and reinfection.

Complications

In areas of the world in which *S. haematobium* infection is commonplace and in which severe and repeated infections occur, the incidence of vesical cancer is high, and is found at a younger age than is normally expected. In contrast to the normal bladder cancer, which is transitional in type, the cancer associated with schistosomiasis is always of squamous type. The aetiology is as yet unknown. Various hypotheses have been suggested to explain the carcinogenic effect of the parasite. These include—

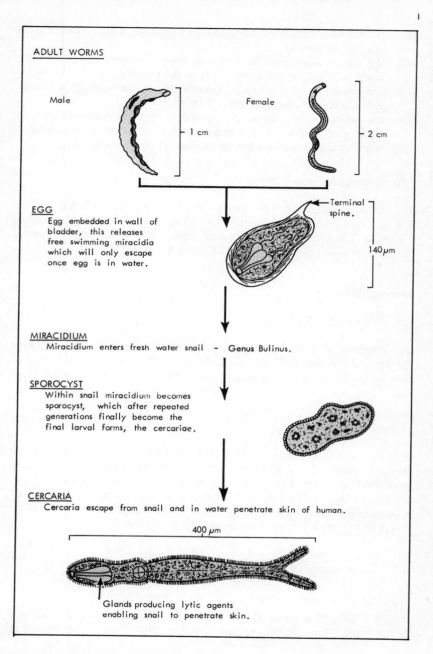

ADULT WORMS

Male   Female

1 cm   2 cm

EGG

Egg embedded in wall of bladder, this releases free swimming miracidia which will only escape once egg is in water.

Terminal spine.

140 μm

MIRACIDIUM

Miracidium enters fresh water snail – Genus Bulinus.

SPOROCYST

Within snail miracidium becomes sporocyst, which after repeated generations finally become the final larval forms, the cercariae.

CERCARIA

Cercaria escape from snail and in water penetrate skin of human.

400 μm

Glands producing lytic agents enabling snail to penetrate skin.

Fig 2.14   Life cycle of Schistosoma haematobium

(a)   the alkaline nature of the cystitis which always accompanies schistosomal infection;

(b)   the mechanical, chronic, irritative effect of the eggs, particularly when calcified, in the deeper parts of the mucosa;

(c)   the possibility of a miracidial toxin acting on the mucosa, particularly if the eggs are trapped but still viable;

(d)   the action of the enzyme glucuronidase on some undefined carcinogenic glucuronide. This enzyme has been shown to be present in schistosomal infections due to its production by the miracidia.

Clinical presentation and diagnosis

The major symptom of infection by the *S. haematobium* is haematuria. This is often associated with the symptoms of cystitis due to secondary infection. The onset of bladder cancer does little to alter the nature of the symptoms but merely exaggerates them.

Investigations

(a)   *Examination of the urine*

The diagnosis of *S. haematobium* is easily made by searching the urine for the eggs of the worm. These have a characteristic appearance, the hook of this particular species being in a terminal position on the somewhat ovoid egg.

(b)   *Cystoscopy*

This may reveal a number of changes according to the degree and duration of the infection. These include hyperaemia, oedema, granulations, ulceration, fine sandy patches, polypi, or carcinoma. A biopsy should be performed on any visible lesion. If the specimen is positive, the eggs will be seen surrounded by varying degrees of reaction and, of course, in the latter stages of the disease squamous cancer may be identified.

(c)   *Intravenous pyelography*

A variety of deviations from normal may be seen including—

(i)   filling defects on the cystogram which are due to the acute proliferating granulomatous lesions, blood clot, or to actual carcinoma;

(ii)   hydronephrosis caused either by obstructive lesions of the lower ureters or contraction of the bladder;

(iii) gross calcification of the bladder and lower ureters;
(iv) non-functioning kidneys.

Treatment

In young patients the schistosomal granulation tissue may resolve under a variety of antischistosomal drugs which include niridazole, metrifonate and the antimonials and which bring relief from obstruction, resolution of hydronephrosis and, in some patients, a return to normal renal function.

Usually, surgery is required only when there is chronic or repeated infection; it is directed towards the relief of obstruction. Once carcinomatous degeneration has occurred the disease is commonly inoperable and resort must be made to radiotherapy or chemotherapy, but whatever the treatment the prognosis is exceedingly poor.

SCHISTOSOMA MANSONI

Life cycle

The life cycle of *S. mansoni* is similar to that of *S. haematobium* excepting that the ova of the former are deposited in the venules of the inferior mesenteric vein so that the subsequent pathological lesions develop in the large bowel.

Pathology

The pathological lesions caused by *S. mansoni* are very similar to those of *S. haematobium* in that granulomata and papilloma form in the bowel wall, after which mucosal ulceration leads to secondary infection and eventually the bowel wall increases in thickness due to advancing fibrosis. Strictures, however, rarely occur.

Malignant degeneration

It is still in doubt whether *S. mansoni* can induce malignant change. The conclusions of various authorities have been somewhat different. Shindo (1976), who reviewed 276 cases of adenocarcinoma of the colon associated with schistosomal infection, found a significant difference between it and carcinoma unassociated with such infection in regard to age, sex ratio, symptoms and histopathological findings, and suggested in consequence that the schistosome could induce malignancy.

Clinical presentation

Symptoms

The initial symptoms associated with *S. mansoni* are commonly inter-mittent abdominal pain and attacks of mucus diarrhoea. When there has been mucosal ulceration, blood and pus are found in the stools and the clinical picture resembles ulcerative colitis, which is an extremely un-common disease in the native African, or carcinoma of the colon, which is also rare because of the relatively low age at death, or lastly, amoebic colitis, which is common.

Signs

Physical examination may reveal the easily palpable thickened loops of bowel, and if the rectum is severely involved, rectal prolapse may occur or fistula in ano.

In severe cases the ova are carried in the portal system to the liver, in which periportal fibrosis develops, later to be followed by portal hyper-tension (*see Tutorials in Surgery: 1,* page 198). Portal hypertension is naturally accompanied by increasing splenomegaly.

Surgical treatment

Surgical treatment is usually reserved for those cases in which medical treatment fails to halt the progress of the disease and bowel complications have occurred. Portal hypertension may demand surgical treatment if bleeding occurs from the enlarging oesophageal varices.

SCHISTOSOMA JAPONICUM (Katayama disease)

S. japonicum mainly affects the small bowel and the proximal part of the large bowel. The pathological changes are similar to those found after infection with *S. mansoni* but tend to be more severe and extensive be-cause of the greater number of ova produced by this parasite. Changes also occur at an early stage in the liver and spleen and the mesentery and omentum become so thickened and fibrotic that they may so constrict the colon that the intestine becomes obstructed.

3   AMOEBIASIS

Causative agent

The protozoa, *Entamoeba histolytica* is small, measuring 10 to 40 μm. On a warm stage, the cell is constantly active erupting from the surface pseudopodia which contain a hyaline cytoplasm. In the living cell little intracellular detail can be made out although, in a case of active dysentery, ingested red cells can be recognised within the parasite.

Life cycle (Fig. 2.15)

Primary development occurs in the lumen of the large intestine in which the amoebae thrive, feeding on bacteria and reproducing by binary fusion. Invasion of the mucosa leads to necrosis and ulceration and from this site the protozoa may spread to form abscesses in other tissues, particularly the liver, and less commonly in the lung or brain.

In favourable conditions the amoebae encyst. A living cyst has the appearance under the microscope of an air bubble or oil droplet. Within it there may be small retractile rods, the chromatoid bodies, which are thought to be aggregations of ribosomes, and, on reaching maturity, four nuclei.

The cysts are passed in the faeces of the host and may remain viable for several weeks. Once ingested the cyst becomes active, and in the small intestine the contained cytoplasm begins to squeeze through the cyst wall until the whole amoeba is finally free in the lumen. At this point each of the four nuclei divide, followed by the cell itself, so that eight small amoebae are produced from a single cyst. Amoebae passed in the stools survive only for two or three days and are not infective because they are destroyed in the stomach.

Distribution

Amoebiasis is of world-wide distribution and infection in man is nearly always contracted from a human source, the infection spreading from man to man by the faecal-oral route. The disease is commonly spread by carriers who themselves have few or no symptoms and who may give no history whatsoever of a previous attack of dysentery.

The spread of infection is linked to factors such as poor personal hygiene, food handling by carriers, and contamination of food by flies or, in the case of uncooked vegetables, the use of human excreta as fertiliser.

The relationship between the parasite and clinical dysentery is, however, unclear. The large *E. histolytica,* indigenous in Britain although morphologically identical with the invasive tropical strains, is non-

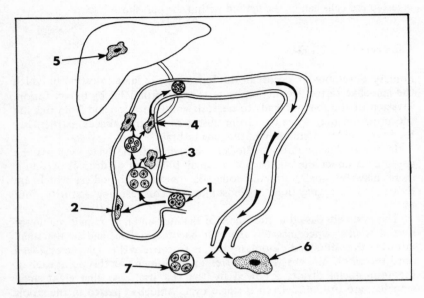

Fig 2.15   Life cycle of Entamoeba histolytica
1. Swallowed cyst about to enter colon   2. Invasive amoeba producing ulceration of wall
of bowel   3. Commensal amoeba   4. Invasive amoeba passing into portal blood stream
5. Amoebic abscess filled with "anchovy sauce"   6. Trophozoite which dies   6. Cyst
capable of infecting further individuals

pathogenic. Some strains appear to be more invasive than others and it has been suggested that the bacterial flora of the gut may predispose to invasion of the mucosa.

INTESTINAL AMOEBIASIS

Pathology

Penetration of the intestinal mucosa by the trophozoite is followed by ulceration, most commonly in the caecum, sigmoid colon, and rectum. The parasite, having penetrated the mucosa, appears to spread in the submucosal tissue rather than in the mucosa itself, producing the classic 'flask-shaped' lesion. In the absence of secondary infection little more than a mild mononuclear reaction occurs. Occasionally, bacterial infection causes the formation of a granulomatous lesion known as an amoeboma, or perforation of the bowel which leads to a localised pericolic abscess or general peritonitis.

Clinical presentation

The intestinal symptoms of amoebiasis depend upon the severity of the infection. When mild, the patient may only complain of intermittent abdominal pain associated with the passage of three or four loose stools a day. Little may be found on clinical examination other than tenderness, particularly in the right side of the abdomen. Severer infections cause blood as well as mucus in the stools. Such attacks may last for days or weeks before a remission, and at any time an acute exacerbation associated with severe bloody diarrhoea and tenesmus or perforation followed by peritonitis and death may occur. The clinical features, therefore, of acute intestinal amoebiasis are very similar to those of acute non-specific ulcerative colitis *but* it should be remembered that in areas in which amoebiasis is common, colitis is rare.

Should an amoeboma develop, clinical examination reveals a mass, usually in the right side of the abdomen. This must be distinguished from conditions such as ileocaecal tuberculosis, Crohn's disease, and carcinoma of the caecum.

Diagnosis

(a) Sigmoidoscopy

The classic sigmoidoscopic appearance of amoebic colitis is one of discrete mucosal ulceration. Each ulcer produces a slight elevation of the mucosa accompanied by a small central depression which contains a minute slough. When the disease is limited to the caecum and ascending colon no sigmoidoscopic evidence of disease will be seen.

(b)   *Stool examination*

Specimens of fresh stools should be repeatedly examined on a warm stage. The presence of cysts does not constitute proof that the symptoms are the result of amoebiasis since carriers of the disease are not uncommon.

(c)   *Serological tests*

Complement fixation tests and gel diffusion techniques can now be performed using a cultured *E. histolytica* as the antigen. A positive result indicates invasive amoebiasis but a negative result does not exclude the disease.

(d)   *Therapeutic trial*

When sigmoidoscopy and stool examination are negative but there is adequate reason to suspect amoebiasis, a short course of emetine can be administered. The diagnosis is positive if improvement occurs within six days of starting treatment.

(e)   *Radiological diagnosis*

This examination is usually reserved for patients in whom a palpable mass is found in the right side of the abdomen. A filling defect resembling either carcinoma or ileocaecal tuberculosis may be seen.

Treatment

(a)   *Medical*

The treatment of intestinal amoebiasis requires the use of a drug which attacks the amoebae in the lumen of the gut and is, therefore, relatively insoluble, and a second drug which, carried in the blood stream, attacks the trophozoite in the wall of the gut. A number of drugs are now available, including emetine and the iodinated quinolones, diloxamide and di-iodohydronyquinoline.

(b)   Indications for surgical intervention

Uncomplicated intestinal amoebiasis never requires surgical treatment. However, the development of an amoeboma or acute fulminating disease occasionally necessitates resection. Such operations must be accompanied by concurrent intensive anti-amoebic therapy.

Severe haemorrhage or perforation may necessitate the use of surgical resection, performing either total colectomy, together with immediate ileorectal anastomosis, or a total colectomy and ileostomy, leaving the rectal stump in situ for future restoration of bowel continuity.

HEPATIC AMOEBIASIS

Pathology

In severe infections the amoebae invade the portal system and are carried to the liver. If these are few in number each amoebic embolus becomes surrounded by an acute inflammatory reaction, and death of the invading trophozoites occurs. During this period the liver may swell and become tender.

When, however, large numbers of amoebae reach the liver, some survive, multiply and produce liquefaction. The liquified and necrotic liver tissue form the so-called 'amoebic abscess' which is not, in fact, a true abscess because it contains no pus. The feebleness of the inflammatory response may lead to rapid enlargement of the cavity which is surrounded by relatively little fibrosis. Approximately 80 per cent of amoebic abscesses develop in the right lobe of the liver, possibly because blood from the right side of the colon flows into this lobe. The contents of a mature amoebic abscess are classically described as 'anchovy sauce' because of the necrotic liver tissue within the cavity.

Invasion of the liver produces tenderness and enlargement of the organ but if the infection is limited, it will be defeated and the organ will return to normal within a few days.

If an amoebic 'abscess' develops, there is fever and the liver enlarges rapidly but jaundice only occurs if a large intrahepatic bile duct is occluded.

The chief danger associated with an amoebic abscess is the frequency with which rupture may occur. This may then be complicated by the development of an empyema or lung abscess, generalised peritonitis, or the development of a communication between the abscess cavity and the biliary tract, the skin or the colon.

Examination usually reveals a hepatomegaly, a high, swinging fever and night sweats.

Diagnosis

(a) *Chest X-ray.* This may demonstrate a raised immobile diaphragm, some collapse of the lung, and a pleural effusion.

(b) *Blood count.* A polymorphonuclear leucocytosis is always present.

(c) *Liver scan.* A filling defect in the liver will be present if an abscess has become established.

(d) *Aspiration.* This diagnostic measure is now less frequently used than in the past. It is normally performed under local anaesthesia using a wide bore needle mounted on a syringe with a two-way tap. A successful aspirate reveals the typical anchovy sauce contents of the cavity.

Treatment

The majority of abscesses respond to treatment with metrinidazole or emetine, and in areas in which amoebiasis is commonplace early medical treatment rather than repeated attempts at aspiration is now the treatment of choice.

4   ASCARIASIS

Infection with the round worm, *Ascaris lumbricoides,* can cause surgical complications.

Life cycle

The life cycle of this worm is extraordinary. The larvae emerging from the eggs that have been swallowed by man burrow into the intestinal mucosa and are then carried by the blood stream to reach the capillaries of the pulmonary circulation. Here they moult to the third stage, and after a short time burst into the alveoli where they undergo a further moult. The larvae, now in the fourth stage, migrate upwards in the bronchial tree and finally reach the back of the throat where they are once more carried down into the digestive tract by the simple act of swallowing. In the small intestine they undergo one final moult to become adult worms some 10 to 20 cm long. The eggs produced by the adult female can live for a considerable period of time after being passed in the faeces and are able to withstand disposal in advanced sewage systems, desiccation, and low temperatures.

Clinical presentation

The presence of a few worms has probably little or no effect on general health. However, during the passage of a large crop of larvae through the lungs, a cough, bronchospasm and eosinophilia may occur and plain radiographs of the chest may show the presence of multiple, soft, mottled opacities.

Of greater importance to the surgeon is the mechanical effect of a bolus formed by a large number of worms entwining, which may result in intestinal obstruction. Furthermore, the adult worms tend to migrate and their entry into the common bile duct may result in biliary obstruction, jaundice and even a suppurative cholangitis, while migration into the pancreatic duct may result in acute pancreatitis. Once lodged in these ducts the worm usually dies and may even become calcified.

Treatment

Although the roundworm can be killed by the piperazine salts reinfection is commonplace in areas in which personal hygiene is poor. Surgery is required to deal with obstruction or to remove dead worms lodged in the common bile or pancreatic ducts.

5   FILARIASIS

The filarial worms of greatest importance to man include the *Wucheria bancrofti* and *Brugia malayi* which cause elephantiasis and Loa loa, the eye worm. The former are widely distributed in tropical areas although the distribution of the worms is limited by the vectors, i.e. the mosquito.

Life cycle

The adult nematodes of *W. bancrofti* live in the lymphatic system in which the female lays the first stage larvae enclosed in an elongated eggshell. The larvae migrate via the lymphatic system to the blood stream where they can inadvertently infect the mosquito which is the intermediate host. In the arthropod, the larvae develop in the haemacele of the labium and when the mosquito bites, the larvae emerge and enter the wound. Once within man the parasite completes its development by moulting twice and migrating through the tissues into the lymphatic system, there to produce the first stage larvae, or microfilarae approximately one year after infection.

Clinical presentation

The adult nematodes spend their lives in the lymph nodes of the body but most commonly affect those of the inguinal region in which, by their presence, they cause a slowly progressive sclerosing inflammation which ultimately causes obstruction of the lymphatics and, therefore, lymph-oedema, popularly called elephantiasis.

Prior to the development of elephantiasis the affected nodes are enlarged, rubbery, and painless. Although the lower limb is commonly involved, other parts of the body are occasionally affected. The scrotum and its contents may be affected, the scrotal skin may become thickened, bilateral hydroceles and bilateral epididymitis may occur.

Any affected area is liable to secondary bacterial infection, usually with the Streptococcus, the repeated attacks of infection hastening the onset of lymphoedema and producing attacks of so-called 'filarial fever'.

Diagnosis

The disease should be suspected by the presence of the rubbery hard lymph nodes. Confirmation may be obtained by the identification of microfilaria in the blood, specimens of which should be taken at night during which period the larval forms flood into the peripheral circulation; they withdraw into the pulmonary capillaries and great veins by day. It is possible to identify the microfilariae in a wet specimen or, alternatively, they can be stained by Leishman or Giemsa's stain.

2.11 THE MANAGEMENT OF BURNS AND SCALDS

Factors that increase the incidence of burns and scalds.

1   *Age*

(*a*)   In the majority of children under three years of age the injury is a scald, caused either by a hot-water bottle bursting in the cot, or the accidental tipping over of a pan or kettle containing boiling water onto an infant.

(*b*)   After the child has learned to walk a large percentage of burns are caused by 'backing-up' against an open coal or gas fire when wearing inflammable night attire.

(*c*)   During an adult's working life the majority of burns are the result of industrial accidents.

(*d*)   In adults over 60 years of age, momentary blackouts based upon cerebral atherosclerosis or arterial spasm become common.

2   *Disease*

(*a*)   Epilepsy.
(*b*)   Cerebral atherosclerosis.
(*c*)   Alcoholism.

3   *Occupation*

Individuals dealing with industrial processes requiring heat are liable to burns or scalds, e.g. foundry workers or laundry workers. Regardless of their cause the two important problems in the management of burns and scalds are (*a*) resuscitation, and (*b*) the treatment of the resulting wound.

1   **RESUSCITATION**

Factors affecting resuscitation

The need for resuscitation and the type of fluid that is required is determined by—
(*a*)   the area of the burn or scald,
(*b*)   the depth of the burn.

(*a*)   *The area*

The area of a burn or scald is of great importance because it determines the volume of the fluid and protein loss.

The area affected can be assessed from the rule of nine, first devised by Polaski and Tennison but often referred to as Wallace's rule. This divides the body surface into areas, the head and neck being equal to 9 per cent of the total body surface, the anterior surface of the trunk 18 per cent, the posterior surface 18 per cent, each lower extremity 18 per cent, each upper extremity 9 per cent, and the perineum 1 per cent. Note that the surface of an individual's hand with the fingers extended is equal to 1 per cent of the body surface of an adult. Although this rule is accurate enough for clinical purposes it is actually not a true measurement of the areas of the various parts of the body since the percentage covered by each, changes relative to another as growth occurs. Thus, the relative surface area of the thigh and leg increases with growth whereas that of the head and face decreases.

In a child, the critical area is usually considered to be 9 per cent and in the adult 18 per cent. If the area involved is greater than this, intravenous therapy should be provided as soon as possible to prevent the onset of hypovolaemic shock since immediately the burn or scald is sustained plasma-like fluid begins to leak from the affected surface. Some of this may appear on the surface to be temporarily contained in blisters while the majority leaks from the damaged capillaries into the interstitial tissues in which it is sequestrated. This loss is greatest in the first 24 hours and comes to an end within 48 hours; in an adult, approximately 1 litre of plasma is lost for every 10 per cent of the body surface burnt or scalded.

(b)   The depth

The depth of a burn or scald is also important in terms of resuscitation for two main reasons—
1   The depth determines the magnitude of red cell loss. This is because:
(a)   the deeper the burn the greater the degree of haemolysis of the erythrocytes following their direct exposure to heat;
(b)   of the greater entrapment of red cells by thrombosis in blood vessels within the area of the burn;
(c)   the morphology of the erythrocytes passing through the damaged area is so altered that they are subsequently sequestrated and prematurely destroyed;
(d)   red cells are lost by sludging.
The magnitude of the erythrocyte destruction in severe burns can often be appreciated from the appearance of free haemoglobin in the blood and urine.

2   Loss of skin leads to increased water loss from the body surface by evaporation. Normally, this loss in a temperate climate is approximately equal to 15 ml/m^2/h whereas in the presence of a full thickness burn it may rise to some 200 ml/m^2/h. This evaporative water loss is accompanied by a corresponding heat loss, each 1 g of water evaporated from the body surface representing a loss of approximately 0.575 kcal. Since the evaporated water is virtually sodium-free, an underestimation of the rate of loss may rapidly end in the development of hypertonic dehydration, hypernatraemia (*see Tutorials in Surgery I,* p. 17.)
Other indications, of course, that resuscitation is required would be—

(a)   a deterioration in the general condition of the patient;
(b)   a rising pulse rate;
(c)   a falling blood pressure;
(d)   a fall in the urine output.
(In all burns or scalds in which intravenous fluids are considered necessary an indwelling catheter should be inserted into the bladder and the hourly volume of urine measured);
(e)   a rising haemocrit.

The last item, of course, indicates the degree of haemoconcentration consequent on the plasma loss and was at one time the keystone to many methods of calculating the volume of plasma necessary to restore a normal circulating blood volume.

Fluid replacement

Three types of fluid can be used to replace the exudate—

1   *Simple or modified saline solutions*

This method has been strongly advocated by Moyer and has many protagonists. In the United Kingdom, the Birmingham Burns Unit tested this method of replacement in children and adults and concluded that it was only satisfactory so long as the patient was closely supervised in the shock period in order that a change to plasma infusion could, if necessary, be made.

2   *Plasma*

This has the advantage of closely resembling the composition of the burn exudate, except in regard to the globulin fraction. The potential disadvantage is that unless 'small pool' plasma is used, transmission of homologous serum jaundice is possible.

3   *The Dextrans*

The dextrans are polysaccharides produced by the fermentation of sucrose by Leuconostoc mesenteroides. Two are in common use as plasma substitutes; dextran 70 and 110. Approximately 40 per cent of the former is lost through the kidneys within 24 hours, but the latter, because it has a larger molecule (average molecular weight 110 000) stays in the circulation for a longer period.

Practice in the United Kingdom. Plasma is most frequently used as replacement fluid in the UK and many formulae have been devised to calculate the volume required. The formula proposed by Muir and Barclay is adequate. First, the area burnt or scalded is assessed by Wallace's rule of nine.

It should be remembered that the period of greatest exudative loss, as previously stated, is within the first 36 hours, but even within this interval the loss is greatest in the first twelve hours. The total period, therefore, is divided into six, of 4, 4, 4, 6, 6 and 12 hours duration respectively. For each period the volume required is the same and can be calculated from the simple formula

$$\frac{Percentage\ area\ of\ body\ burnt \times wt\ in\ kg}{2}$$

The first aliquot of plasma must be transfused within the first four hours and, even if the transfusion does not begin until, say, three hours after burning, the calculated total volume required should be given in the remaining hour.

141

In addition to plasma, 100 ml of water hourly should be given by mouth if the patient does not find it nauseating, or intravenously if oral feeding is impossible.

Furthermore, if the burn is larger than 10 per cent of the total surface area, blood is necessary in addition to plasma, the amount required being equal to 1 per cent of the patient's blood volume for each 1 per cent of the burn area. The approximate blood volume can be calculated from the following simple formula:

$$\text{Blood volume} = \text{Wt in kg} \times 75$$

After the theoretical requirements have been calculated a number of other factors should be considered. Note should be taken that young children and elderly adults will not tolerate excessive quantities of fluid, that patients with pre-existing cardiovascular or renal disease should be treated with caution, and that in flash burns, in which respiratory tract irritation may be present, pulmonary oedema is commonplace. Furthermore, extensive burns are often followed by paralytic ileus and in these patients fluids should not be given by mouth until bowel sounds return.

Assessment of Resuscitation

Clinical evidence suggesting that resuscitation is progressing satisfactorily is provided by the following clinical data—
(a) the patient is calm;
(b) peripheral circulation is adequate;
(c) blood pressure is normal;
(d) pulse rate remains steady;
(e) urine output is satisfactory.

In a child this should be 7 ml/h or more, and in the adult 25 ml/h or more. The urine should be routinely tested for haem pigments because organic renal failure seldom occurs if there are no haem pigments in the urine but if there are, renal failure is possible.

If the urine output falls, the urine specific gravity should be measured because this gives a rough idea of renal concentrating power. In addition, the urine urea and plasma urea concentrations should, if possible, be frequently assessed. Assuming that hypovolaemia has been adequately corrected and oliguria persists a test transfusion of mannitol should be given (see Tutorials in Surgery I, page 16).

DEPTH OF BURN OR SCALD

Although the depth of burn is not an immediate problem, it is essential that it should be accurately assessed as soon as possible since partial thickness burns spontaneously heal within three weeks, whereas burns involving the whole thickness of the skin will usually require the application of a graft.

Unfortunately, at present there is no agreed standard international classification of the depth of burning. The National Research Council of Canada in 1942 simplified what had been a somewhat complex situation by recognising only two degrees of burning—

1 Partial thickness loss, which implies that the deeper epithelial elements are alive and that epithelialisation will take place without grafting.

2 Full thickness loss, which implies that there has been complete destruction of all epithelial elements. Such a burn cannot heal from surface elements but only by the ingrowth of epithelium from the peripheral margin, aided, possibly, by contraction.

Interestingly enough this classification corresponds to that used by Giovanni di Vigo some 500 years earlier.

A much more sophisticated classification based on the skin elements from which a burn may heal has been proposed by Jackson and others of the Birmingham Accident Hospital's Burn Unit. The classification requires an elementary knowledge of the structure of normal skin and takes account of the following five principles—

1 it is based upon the depth of necrosis, not on the intensity of surface burning;
2 it should relate the depth of burning to the critical plane of the deepest epithelial elements;
3 the type of burn should be capable of early diagnosis;
4 the classification should have a prognostic significance indicating:
   (a) whether skin grafting will be necessary;
   (b) the probable type of scarring.
5 the classification should include all the depths of burning commonly distinguished and referred to in clinical practice.

To apply a classification that obeys these five principles requires an elementary knowledge of the normal structure of skin (Fig. 2.16). With the exception of some special sites, which include the scalp, beard, palms and soles, the undersurface of the dermis is composed of a deeper layer of collagenous fibres that cross each other to form an extensive feltwork of rhomboid meshes in which the main direction of the fibres runs parallel with the skin. Through the mesh formed by the fibrous septa, fat from the subcutaneous tissues proper bulges up into the deeper layers of the corium to form domes of varying height. The two specialised elements of the skin, the hair follicles and sweat glands, take origin at different depths; the former arise in the lower dermis and at the very most merely penetrate the summit of the fat domes, whereas the sweat glands penetrate more deeply so that many of them take origin deep in the fat domes even below the level of the rhomboid network of collagen fibres. Some distance deep to the sweat glands is the horizontal, subdermal arterial and venous plexus.

So far as a burn or scald is concerned, any burn that still leaves the remnants of most of the hair follicles and sweat ducts can heal, if properly treated, in about 14 days, whereas if all the hair follicles are destroyed, but a full complement of sweat glands remains, healing will require 21

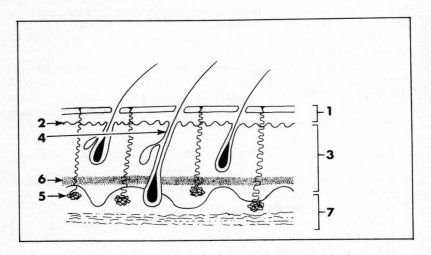

Fig 2.16   Schematic representation of skin structure (After Jackson)
1. Epidermis   2. Stratum germinativum   3. Dermis   4. Hair follicle   5. Sweat gland
6. Level of pain perceiving nerve endings   7. Subdermal plexus

days. Burns deeper than this but still possessing some sweat gland remnants can heal of themselves but the process will be slower. This type of burn has been termed the deep dermal burn, and anything deeper than this in which all epithelial elements have been destroyed is full thickness.

Jackson's classification of burns based on the depth of necrosis is given in Table 2.1.

TABLE 2.1

1	Erytherma	No loss of epidermis	Hyperalgesia
2	Partial thickness skin loss;		
	Superficial	No loss of dermis	Hyperalgesia
	Intermediate	Healing from hair follicles	Normal or hypoalgesic
	Deep	Healing from sweat glands	Hypo or analgesic
3	Deep Dermal Burns	Scanty epithelial foci which may or may not epithelialize the surface under the conditions prevailing	Analgesia
4	Whole skin loss	Healing form edge only	Analgesia

Partial skin loss although easily divisible into three subgroups on anatomical grounds cannot easily be distinguished immediately after burning, and this is so also for the deep dermal burn, the various levels of burning becoming apparent only with the passage of time.

A full thickness burn may, however, be readily diagnosed, the presence of exposed fat, muscle or bone in the depth of the burn leaving no doubt of its severity, as also does the more common brown, somewhat translucent appearance of the skin traversed by thrombosed veins. Simple erythema, with or without blister formation, usually indicates a partial thickness burn, but it should be remembered that the more extensive the burn the more likely it is that some parts will be full thickness. The manner of burning is also important; direct contact with molten metal or boiling fluids nearly always results in full-thickness injury.

Although many attempts have been made to 'map' full-thickness burns, usually by methods designed to investigate the integrity of the blood flow through the burnt area, no method has been universally successful or acceptable.

One clinical test of burn depth is pin-prick sensation, the importance of which was first described by Dupuytren in 1832. The sign is applicable to all patients above the age of three so long as they are co-operative. The appreciation of pin-prick as pain does not disappear until there is necrosis in a plane just superficial to the deepest sweat ducts. Deep partial thickness burns (Jackson's classification) are associated with a reduction in sensation or analgesia; deep dermal burns and full-thickness burns are totally analgesic.

To perform the test properly the skin should be pricked firmly, in several places to the square inch, to be sure that analgesia is present. If the appreciation of pin-prick is sharp, healing will occur within three weeks with no loss of skin texture. If the burn is analgesic, the slough will separate between the 16th to 18th day and a skin graft will be required when the granulation tissue is 'mature'.

BURN DRESSING

1   Occlusive

This method may be used for any burn. If occlusive dressings are applied it is essential that the chemical used on the dressing should neither macerate the tissues nor damage any viable epithelium. Many different antibiotics, either alone or in combination, have been tried. Recently, silver nitrate and silver sulphadiazine have been introduced. The advantage of the latter is that it prevents early invasion of the burn by *Pseudomonas aeruginosa*. After the maximum exudative period is over the dressings can be left undisturbed for periods of between three to five days. Superficial burns heal within 10 to 20 days. Ungrafted deep dermal burns, in the absence of infection, may heal within 25 to 30 days. Full-thickness burns may be excised and grafted forthwith at about 14 days. Whatever the antibacterial compound used a burn dressing should isolate the burn from the environment, and be absorptive and bulky enough to be sure that exudate does not reach the surface.

2   Exposure

This method of treatment is ideal for superficial burns, for burns of the face, or burns involving only one aspect of the circumference of a limb. Normally, prior to exposure the burn is cleansed. The exudate of a partial thickness burn dries in 48 to 72 hours, forming a crust under which epithelial regeneration occurs, and in 14 to 21 days the crust separates spontaneously, leaving an unscarred well-healed surface.

With a full thickness burn the dead tissue becomes a dehydrated thick tough eschar which may slowly separate at the edges or crack across its surface, indicating the need for excision followed by grafting.

TREATMENT OF THE BURN

1   Small full-thickness burns

Burns produced by direct contact with a hot object, molten metal, electrical heating element, or flame, can be excised and grafted as soon as they are first seen.

There are four possible ways of managing the larger burn:

1   Extensive excision

Extensive excision and immediate grafting of whole-thickness burns soon after injury have been subjected to extensive trial in many different centres in the hope that such radical treatment would reduce the mortality. This has not been achieved and the method has been abandoned.

2   Tangential excision followed by immediate grafting (Fig. 2.17)

This technique was initially described by Janzekovic in 1968 and has now been widely adopted when examination of the burn shows that analgesia to pin-prick is present. The presence of analgesia indicates that the burn must, according to Jackson's classification, be partial thickness, at the very least involving the nerve plexus conveying pain, deep dermal or whole thickness.

The two advantages of tangential excision are—

(*a*) If it is found that the subdermal veins are black in colour and obviously thrombosed the surgeon is immediately able to appreciate that the burn involves the whole thickness of the skin and that the excision must be carried deeper before the application of a skin graft.

(*b*) If the reverse is the case and the burn is more superficial than was expected, no harm will come of the procedure because the whole purpose of tangential excision is to leave the deeper parts of the skin with its contained sweat ducts, and if the burn proves to be more superficial than the base of the hair follicles then healing will naturally occur within three weeks.

Technique

(*a*)   Perform between the second and fifth days following injury, having first eliminated *Streptococcus pyogenes* (Group A β-haemolytic strepto-coccus) infection by the prior administration of an appropriate antibio⊹'c such as erythromycin. The other serious infection by *Ps. aeruginosa* does not normally present a problem within the first week following burning.

(*b*)   Map out the area of total analgesia prior to the anaesthetic and then, following anaesthesia, with a Braithwaite knife set to give a fine cut, begin to remove tangential slices of skin, starting from the centre of the burn which is most likely to be the deepest part of the burnt area.

(*c*)   As the slices reach the deeper parts of the dermis it will become obvious whether the subdermal plexus is thrombosed; if this is so, the area should be excised with a scalpel until a suitable graft bed has been produced.

147

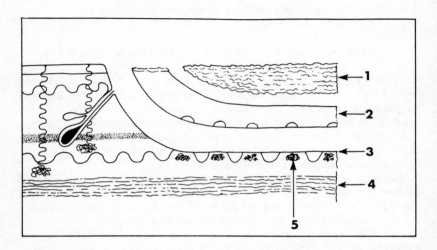

Fig 2.17   Schematic drawing to represent tangenital excision for a deep dermal burn
1. First slice through burn   2. Second slice through burn   3. Base on which skin graft
will be laid   4. Subdermal plexus remains intact, stasis but not thrombosis   5. Sweat
gland remnants

(*d*)   When no thrombosed veins are visible and the tangential excision has reached the fat domes, or a little above, the case can be considered suitable for grafting. At this point, if the procedure has not been carried out under a tourniquet the dermis will be pink in colour and multiple bleeding points will be seen.

(*e*)   The extent of the analgesic area submitted to excision at any one sitting is determined by the availability of blood and donor skin. The latter is particularly important because the graft must be placed on the excised dermis at once, otherwise, if the area is left exposed, the residual dermis will slough.

The donor skin should be a thin razor graft (Fig. 2.18) and the graft should be placed edge-to-edge with no intervening bare area.

(*f*)   A normal take can be assumed if the graft appears pink between the second and third day. If the graft fails to take it probably means that it has been put on a bed that has too great a thickness of ischaemic dermis.

(*g*)   Following the completion of the operation a dressing is applied, the one described by Jackson being tulle gras soaked in neomycin and chlorhexidine, external to which is a layer of cottonwool moistened in 0.5 per cent silver nitrate, and, finally, a crepe bandage.

3   Partial thickness burns

The burn is cleansed. Exudation continues throughout the next 48 to 72 hours but as it lessens in volume so it dries on the surface. In this type of burn the resulting eschar lies above the level of the surrounding skin surface, and under this crust epithelial regeneration takes place unless it is impeded by infection or pressure. Normally, the crust falls away between 10 to 21 days, leaving an unscarred well-healed surface.

4   Full thickness burns

When all layers have been destroyed the dead skin becomes a thick tough eschar with its surface lying at the level of the intact skin. As this dries and contracts it shrinks, so that eventually it lies below the surface of the surrounding healthy skin. The eschar slowly loosens, but the speed with which it does so is dependent upon bacterial growth and the natural development of granulation tissue at the interface between eschar and the normal tissues. At some point in time, usually within the first ten days, a decision must be made regarding the definitive treatment. The most common decision is to abandon exposure, if this has been practised, excise the eschar and, after suitable preparation of the granulating surface, apply split thickness grafts.

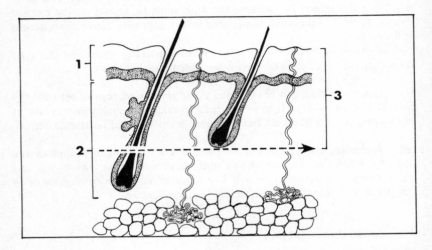

Fig 2.18 Split thickness graft suitable for a burn. Using this type of graft it should be possible to take a second graft in two to three weeks
1. Epidermis   2. Dermis   3. Thickness of skin graft removed

In a child suffering from very extensive burns the principle of 'tiger grafting' can be employed, alternating strips of skin obtained from the mother and the patient. An alternative dressing is pigskin. One advantage of total skin cover, even if this is only temporary, is the reduction of sepsis and the ending of the catabolic phase which is always severe in extensive burns.

NUTRITIONAL SUPPORT

Any severely burnt patient remains in negative nitrogen balance until full skin cover is obtained; furthermore, during the grafting period when frequent loss of blood is sustained care must be taken to maintain the haemoglobin at as near normal levels as possible. To alleviate or diminish the negative nitrogen balance a high calorie diet should be provided, and if necessary the diet should be given by nasogastric tube or, alternatively, by intravenous means. The loss of protein in an adult suffering from a 20 per cent burn may reach 200 g daily; compare this with the loss of 100 g of protein spread over 10 days following cholecystectomy.

In addition to the need for nitrogen, patients suffering from burns are also hypermetabolic so that their calorie requirement is massive, possibly amounting to as much as 10,000 kcal/day.

COMPLICATIONS

1　Immediate

Infection. The burnt area is easily colonised by the ubiquitous *Staphylococcus aureus* and the *Streptococcus pyogenes,* and from about the fifth day onwards by the *Pseudomonas aeruginosa.*

(*a*) Infection with the haemolytic streptococcus has two undesirable side effects. First, it destroys the remaining viable skin cells, thus converting partial skin loss to full thickness, and secondly, it destroys any split thickness skin grafts that may have been applied. A streptococcal infection is usually recognised by the advancing red flare that develops around the burnt area. If the area is already granulating the granulations appear unhealthy.

(*b*) Staphylococcal infection is common but seldom of great clinical importance and, indeed, the *Ps. aeruginosa* may displace it from the burn by the fifth day.

Both streptococcal and staphylococcal infections can be treated by antibiotics in the early period. Penicillin, cloxacillin or clindamycin are all useful, depending on their *in vitro* sensitivity.

(*c*) *Ps. aeruginosa* produces a bluish green pus and proteus infections a foul-smelling pus. The use of silver sulphadiazine delays colonisation with these organisms and, also, the dangers of a Gram-negative septicaemia.

The latter should be recognised by the development of chills, hyperpyrexia, or hyperthermia, tachycardia, tachypnoea, hypotension and the onset of oliguria.

All the hazards of infection are, of course, reduced by early excision and grafting or by tangential excision and grafting, whichever is appropriate, and they have also been reduced by the vast array of available antibiotics. However, the increasing use of antibiotics and the conquest of burn shock have led to fungal infections assuming an increasing importance in burns, the control of which is difficult.

Duodenal and gastric ulceration

This form of peptic ulceration is commonly referred to as Curling's ulcer, the incidence of which increases as the area of the burn increases as demonstrated by routine fibre endoscopy in extensively burned patients. Fibre endoscopy has shown that a large percentage of patients in whom a 30 per cent burn or greater has occurred develop acute erosions in both the stomach and the duodenum and that it is from these acute lesions that penetrating ulceration develops. The development of the latter appears, however, to be related to the pH of the gastric juice and it would seem reasonable to administer cimetidine to all extensive burns in the hope of aborting this complication which may lead to severe upper gastrointestinal bleeding.

Renal failure

Severe burns inadequately resuscitated may be followed by either oliguric or less commonly non-oliguric renal failure.

Liver necrosis

A complication usually following prolonged untreated shock, the typical lesion is a centrilobular haemorrhagic necrosis.

Pulmonary complications

(*a*)　Noxious combustion products might have been inhaled. Physical signs appear in the chest after 24 to 48 hours of injury and, at the same time, derangement in the blood gases develops. If death ensues, post mortem shows congestive oedema and sloughing of the bronchial mucosa.

(*b*)　Pulmonary oedema due to over-loading of the circulation during resuscitation.

(*c*)　Pulmonary atelectasis due to excessive bronchial secretions.

In young children there may be a burn encephalopathy, due to cerebral oedema following resuscitation. Treatment by adrenergic blocking agents, e.g. chlorpromazine, and increased fluid intake and a heat cradle are required. The latter dilates cutaneous vessels and produces increased surface heat loss, so lowering the core temperature which is abnormally high in this condition.

2   **Intermediate complications**

(*a*)   *Pseudomonas aeruginosa* septicaemia;
(*b*)   pneumonic lung changes;
(*c*)   embolic lung phenomena;
(*d*)   *Ducubitus ulcers.* These are a hazard in any extensive burns and can be avoided only by frequent turning;
(*e*)   *Constricting eschar.* This may form if the whole circumference of the limb has been burnt or large areas of the chest wall are involved. The treatment consists of excising part or the whole of the constricting lesion.

3   **Late complications**

(*a*)   *Contractures.* Inevitable contractures follow burns of flexion surfaces or if loose ends such as the eyelid, ear, or lips are involved.
(*b*)   *Hypertrophic scars.* These are particularly liable to follow the spontaneous healing of the deep dermal burn which is one of the reasons for adopting tangential excision and grafting.
(*c*)   *Pruritis.* This is usually a self-limiting complaint but may be exceedingly troublesome.

2.12 DIAGNOSIS AND TREATMENT OF NON-MALIGNANT ANAL CONDITIONS

HAEMORRHOIDS

Classification

External, arising from the skin-covered lower third of the anal canal. *Internal,* arising from the veins of the internal haemorrhoidal plexus in the upper two thirds of the anal canal. Internal haemorrhoids are also divisible into first, second and third degree, according to the degree of prolapse. A third degree pile is one that remains prolapsed after defaecation but can usually be manually replaced. Piles arise in three main areas; situated when looking at the anus with the patient placed in lithotomy, at the 3, 7 and 11 o'clock positions, corresponding to the anatomical position of the main haemorrhoidal vessels.

Aetiological factors

1 Venous engorgement due to obstruction of the portal venous system or local obstruction by a neoplasm of the rectum;
2 Increased intra-abdominal pressure, e.g. pregnancy;
3 Constipation;
4 Lack of support to the haemorrhoidal plexus, which may follow operations that disturb or destroy the sphincter, e.g. operation for the cure of complicated fistulae.

Symptomatology

Social uncleanliness, bleeding, prolapse and pruritis. Occasionally, there may be severe anaemia.

Diagnosis

This requires inspection, digital examination, proctoscopy, and sigmoidoscopy.

External haemorrhoids must be distinguished from a carcinoma of the anal canal. Internal haemorrhoids must be distinguished from a prolapse of the rectum. When the main symptom is bleeding, the differential diagnosis includes proctitis and carcinoma of the rectum.

Treatment

Many treatments for internal haemorrhoids have been described, among these are—

1 *Injection therapy using phenol in almond oil*

Four to five ml is injected into the submucous areolar tissue above each internal haemorrhoid. The effect is to produce a mild inflammatory foreign-body type of response. This form of treatment is most effective when the piles do not prolapse and are not associated with large skin tags.

Complications are uncommon but include—
(a) Ulceration at the site of injection; this does not occur after a single but only after repeated injections.

154

(b)   Chemical prostatitis leading to perineal pain, frequency, and dysuria due to injecting the sclerosant into the prostate.

2   Strangulation by rubber bands

This method has been more frequently used in the United States than in the U.K. It is applicable only to second and third degree haemorrhoids in which the strangulating band can be placed over a definite pedicle.

3   Lord's procedure

In 1969, Lord suggested that internal haemorrhoids were caused by circular constricting bands in the anal canal which, by causing difficulty in defaecation, led to straining at stool and increased venous pressure in the haemorrhoidal plexus. He, therefore, suggested that the condition could be cured if these bands were broken down by severe dilatation of the anal canal. The basis of Lord's procedure is that four fingers of each hand should be inserted as far as possible into the anus. After dilatation, a large sponge is inserted into the anal canal to prevent the development of a haematoma. This is removed once the patient has recovered from the anaesthetic, and postoperatively the patient dilates the anus with a 4-cm diameter perspex dilator, at first daily and then less frequently. Few other surgeons have, however, been able to reproduce the excellent results achieved by Lord himself. The following complications of Lord's procedure have been described; rectal prolapse, continued prolapse of the haemorrhoids, and rectal incontinence.

4   Surgical excision

A variety of different operations have been described for the treatment of second and third degree haemorrhoids. The common operative technique requires dissection of the pile-bearing areas and ligation of the pedicles at the level of the internal sphincter. This operation is particularly associated with the names of Milligan and Morgan. Other well-known procedures include Park's submucous resection and Farquharson's clamp and cautery method. In addition, second and third degree haemorrhoids may be destroyed by freezing with liquid nitrogen, although most exponents of this technique admit to difficulties with the residual skin tags.

Complications of haemorrhoidectomy

Immediate

1 reactionary haemorrhage;
2 pain;
3 retention of urine;
4 secondary haemorrhage.

Delayed

1 loss of sphincter control, which may be sufficient to produce social inconvenience, particularly in times of stress, as in diarrhoea.
2 stricture formation, either internal at a mucosal level or external at skin level.
3 residual skin tags.

Complications of internal haemorrhoids

The most significant complications of internal haemorrhoids are—

1 severe chronic anaemia;
2 prolapse followed by strangulation;
3 thrombosis followed by the development of a fibrous polyp;
4 infection followed by the development of a submucous abscess.

External haemorrhoids, skin tags

These may have no apparent cause but they are often complicated by repeated attacks of thrombosis provoked by an attack of constipation. This causes severe pain or chronic pruritis. The common complaint is lack of hygiene, and the treatment consists of formal excision and ligation if the pile is associated with an internal haemorrhoid.

FISSURE-IN-ANO

This is the commonest cause of severe rectal pain. The condition consists of a longitudinal ulcer lying over and exposing the lower third of the internal sphincter. It is nearly always found in the posterior 6 o'clock position except in women when it may lie anteriorly. The lower end of a fissure is often marked by a fibrous tag known as a 'sentinel' pile. The pain associated with a fissure begins at the time of defaecation and often continues for several hours thereafter. The severity of the pain induces secondary constipation. There may be bleeding, but it is rarely excessive and is usually restricted to a few drops on the toilet paper.

Diagnosis

This principally involves inspection, because all fissures can be seen if sufficient care is taken. Palpation quickly demonstrates the associated anal spasm. When examining a patient complaining of anal pain it is as well to remember that a squamous cell carcinoma of the anal canal or an adeno-carcinoma of the rectum that has infiltrated the anus will produce exactly similar symptoms. Colitis and Crohn's disease are frequently associated with anal and perianal lesions, but they are usually gross, and despite their appearance may cause little pain or discomfort.

Treatment

Conservative

Anaesthetic ointments may be applied before and after defaecation. If healing does not take place within 3 or 4 weeks, operative treatment should be considered.

Surgery

1 The simplest manoeuvre involves gentle dilatation of the anus until it admits four fingers. This simple procedure produces satisfactory relief of pain in nearly all patients, but the sentinel pile remains.

2 *Internal sphincterotomy.* Not until 1953 was it shown by Eisenhammer that sphincterotomy was a division of the internal sphincter. Until that time surgeons had been under the mistaken impression that the operation they were performing for the treatment of a fissure was a division of the external sphincter.

The internal sphincter may be divided from within the anal canal, or by subcutaneous tenotomy from without, and not more than the lower half of the sphincter need be divided. Immediate relief of pain usually follows the operation but the internal wound takes some weeks to heal. Leakage and soiling may be troublesome after sphincterotomy.

FISTULA-IN-ANO

This condition consists of a track lined by granulation tissue leading from the anal canal or lower rectum to the exterior. Frequently, there is only one internal opening, whereas there may be multiple external openings; occasionally, no internal opening actually exists, when the condition should be more nearly defined as a sinus.

Aetiological factors

(*a*) Previous pyogenic abscess. Many of these probably arise as a complication of a fissure in ano but in the absence of such a history Parks *et al,* maintain that in many the initial infection affects the anal ducts or glands which discharge at the muco-cutaneous junction of the anal canal into the anal crypts. The glands pass through the internal sphincter to end in the areolar tissue of the intersphincteric zone at which point they form small glandular structures surrounded by lymphoid tissue. Parks and his colleagues believe that abscesses develop in this intersphincteric plane and from there spread downwards to the anal margin, upwards into the rectal wall, or outwards through the external sphincter into the ischiorectal space.

(b)   *Ulcerative colitis.* 3 to 6 per cent of patients suffering from colitis have associated fistulae.

(c)   *Crohn's disease.* Crohn himself reported this complication in 18 per cent of patients and this incidence has since been confirmed. Fistulae develop more frequently in colonic than small bowel disease.

(d)   Carcinoma of the lower third of the rectum and anal canal.

(e)   Rare conditions leading to fistulae are tuberculosis and actinomycosis.

Anatomical classification of fistulae

Goodsall's rule. The position of the external opening should be noted. Goodsall observed that when the external opening of a fistula lies behind a transverse line drawn across the mid-point of the anus the internal opening is in the midline on the posterior wall of the anal canal. In contrast, when the external opening is anterior to this line the fistula runs directly backwards into the anal canal.

Classification in terms of vertical plane

The most important issue in regard to the vertical height to which the fistula rises is in relationship to the puborectalis muscle. As a general rule the whole of the internal and most of the external sphincter can be divided, with the exception of the puborectalis muscle, without any serious loss of function. This is, however, true only for the younger patient. In an elderly person with a weak external sphincter even partial division of the internal sphincter may cause incontinence, hence the varying degrees of incontinence seen following haemorrhoidectomy.

The most simplistic way of considering fistula-in-ano is to consider them as high or low, depending on the relationship of the internal opening to the levator ani. All high fistulae open at or above this level and are rare, whereas low level fistulae open below. Parks and his colleagues, in their paper in the *British Journal of Surgery*, while recognising the importance of the puborectalis, divide fistulae into four main types—

1 the intersphincteric, when the tract runs between the internal and external sphincters;

2 the trans-sphincteric, when the tract passes through both the internal and external sphincters but below the level of the puborectalis;

3 the suprasphincteric, when the tract beginning in an intersphincteric position runs over the upper border of the puborectalis;

4 the extrasphincteric, when the tract is wholly external to the sphincters or beginning in the intersphincteric position passes laterally and then upwards and down external to the sphincters.

Each of these main types can then, according to their thesis, again be subdivided until finally 13 different types of fistula require consideration. Fortunately for the practising surgeon, 90 per cent of all fistulae lie below the level of the puborectalis and the risk, therefore, of incontinence is minimal in most patients. The most important factor to remember is not to pass a probe or fistula directly upwards through the levator ani and into the rectum when no natural opening exists, since this type of fistula will heal if given free drainage through the ischiorectal fossa.

Symptomatology

There is nearly always a history of previous perianal suppuration. A fistula rarely discharges continuously and, usually after a latent period of days, weeks or months, the patient develops a further painful perianal swelling which later discharges either through the original orifice or by an entirely new one.

Diagnosis

Examination confirms the diagnosis. Sigmoidoscopy rules out the presence of neoplasm, proctocolitis and, possibly, Crohn's disease, after which the most important step is to discover the relationship between the internal opening and the ano-rectal ring that marks the level of the levator ani. In low level anterior fistulae it may be possible to pass a probe through the fistula without an anesthetic, but in most fistulae a 'light' anaesthetic will be required; 'light', at least initially, because it is essential to palpate the muscular fibres of puborectalis.

The diagnosis of fistula is not difficult, but occasionally the condition may be confused with hyperhidrosis suppurativa.

Treatment

The treatment of all fistulae is surgical. The principle of the operation is to lay open the track. In doing so, the greater part of both the external and the internal sphincters may be divided. Great care is required after laying open the track or tracks to make sure that the saucerised wound heals from its depth. The common postoperative complaint is incontinence. In the younger patient this is fortunately only temporary.

2.13 THE COMPLICATIONS OF COLOSTOMY AND ILEOSTOMY

COMPLICATIONS OF COLOSTOMY

1   Early

(a)   *Necrosis* (sloughing)

An important early complication of terminal or end colostomy is necrosis of the bowel wall proximal to the mucocutaneous suture line. The cause of this complication is a poor blood supply brought about either by faulty ligature of blood vessels supplying the gut, or to early thrombosis in arteries or veins that are possibly constricted by the tension exerted on a short loop in the obese patient, or by the external oblique aponeurosis.

If unrecognised, this can be a serious complication because, as the bowel wall sloughs, a coliform and bacteriodes infection of the sub-cutaneous fat may lead to extensive cellulitis and, possibly, gangrene of the abdominal wall.

In most patients the treatment of this condition demands reopening of the original abdominal incision and preparation of a new loop from within.

(b)   *Lateral space obstruction*

This form of early small bowel obstruction was relatively common prior to routine closure of the intraperitoneal space that lies on the lateral side of an end colostomy. Following recognition of this form of obstruction, the space was routinely closed (Fig. 2.19) and the complication became extremely rare. It was finally completely eliminated by the use of the extraperitoneal technique (Fig. 2.20).

However, early small gut obstruction may still come about because of kinking, and obstruction of a small bowel loop on the cut edge of the peritoneum or prolapse through the repaired pelvic peritoneum.

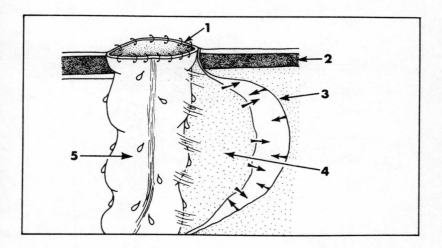

Fig 2.19   Closure of lateral space by suture
1. Direct muco-cutaneous suture   2. Abdominal parietes   3. Peritoneal covering of lateral abdominal wall   4. Mesentery of descending colon united to peritoneum of lateral abdominal wall by either single purse string suture or multiple sutures according to preference of surgeon   5. Sigmoid colon

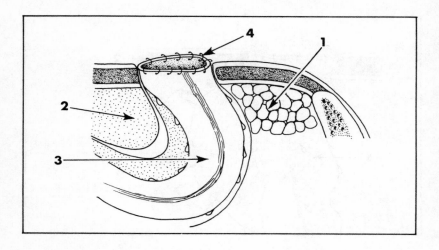

Fig 2.20   Extraperitoneal colostomy
1. Extraperitoneal fat   2. Parietal peritoneum   3. Sigmoid colon   4. Direct mucocutaneous suture

2   Late

(a)   Stenosis

This complication was once the most common after colostomy operations, but following the introduction of immediate direct mucocutaneous stitching it is now rare. When stenosis occurs it can be treated in one of two ways. The stenotic area of skin can be divided and excised, after which the skin and mucosa are resutured. This is a minor procedure which may, if necessary, be performed using local anaesthesia. It will not, however, result in a long-term cure of the condition which can be achieved only by completely refashioning the colostomy. It may be sufficient to excise the skin around the whole circumference of the stoma, then to deepen the dissection, even into the peritoneal cavity, so that the loop can be brought to the surface with plenty of slack, after which a direct mucocutaneous suture is performed. Occasionally, however, refashioning demands reconstruction of the loop from within.

(b)   Herniation

There is nearly always gross herniation if a colostomy is brought out through a major abdominal incision, and it was also common when brought out through a left iliac fossa stab wound. Although minor degrees of herniation are still relatively common, the adoption of extraperitoneal construction has led to the herniae being smaller and less obtrusive.

Massive herniae of long duration may produce sufficient disability to demand repair. This should be approached with caution. Non-absorbable materials are contra-indicated because of the possibilities of infection followed by chronic sinus formation. If the hernia is large, the return of the contents may lead to embarrassment of the cardiorespiratory system or, occasionally, precipitate the development of a sacral hernia.

(c)   Prolapse

This complication is rarely seen following the construction of a terminal colostomy but it is commonplace following loop colostomy, and it is especially troublesome in the neonate, in which the commonest indications for loop colostomy are anorectal agenesis and Hirschsprung's disease. Before considering amputation of the prolapse in an infant the surgeon should remember that this may later lead to great technical difficulties in performing a definitive operation such as the Svenson abdominoanal pull through operation.

Whereas an ileostomy that is continent can be constructed (page 167), it has long been accepted that a colostomy is inevitably incontinent because all the various surgical manoeuvres that have been tried have proved unavailing.

In 1975, however, Feustel and Henning of Erlangen introduced an entirely original idea in the form of a magnetic closing device consisting of a ring and cap, both magnetised. The ring consists of samarium-cobalt coated with an acrylate, which is implanted in the abdominal wall around the emerging colon, and the cap consists of a plastic disc with a central protruding spigot enclosing a samarium-cobalt core.

However, the results published by the originators of this technique in a relatively large series, i.e. 105 patients, showed that the ring had to be removed in about one-fifth of all patients because of sepsis, and that only a quarter were fully continent for both flatus and faeces.

Other surgeons have also had relatively disappointing results following this procedure and it seems probable from the literature that in terms of age and build alone at least 50 per cent of patients should never be considered for the insertion of such a device and that in the remaining patients many would do just as well without this device as with it.

COMPLICATIONS OF ILEOSTOMY

1 Early

Necrosis

If the blood supply to an ileostomy is inadequate, the projecting bowel becomes purple and an offensive serosanguineous discharge occurs instead of the normal early non-offensive fluid motion.

This complication requires immediate exploration and, if necessary, total reconstruction of the ileostomy loop from within the abdomen.

2 Late

(a) Recession

The ideal ileostomy should project 2.5 to 3.5 cm beyond the abdominal wall; it may, however, recede either intermittently or permanently. This relatively common complication is important because severe recession is nearly always associated with difficulties in controlling the ileostomy outflow, part or all of the effluent being discharged at the skin level.

Problems arise with the management of the ileostomy flange which cannot be made to adhere to the moist skin and this almost immediately causes skin excoriation. Treatment is determined by the severity of the condition. When the outflow cannot be managed by conservative means the ileostomy must be reconstructed by means of an intra-abdominal approach.

(b) Stenosis

This complication, which was once common at the skin level, has virtually disappeared following the general use of direct mucocutaneous suture after eversion of the projecting bowel. Before the introduction of this technique by Brookes (1952), stenosis affected approximately 30 per cent of stoma. Rarely, the bowel may be constricted at the level of the parietal peritoneum. An early symptom of ileostomy stenosis is an increase in the volume of the outflow together with intermittent colicky abdominal pain. Severe malfunction may lead to electrolyte and water depletion, and because the discharge is watery, there may be temporary mechanical difficulties with adhesion of the flange. The diagnosis can usually be made by digital examination of the stoma, and confirmed by erect X-rays of the abdomen, which show the classic fluid levels of small-gut obstruction. Internal obstruction requires intra-abdominal correction with the fashioning of a new ileostomy. Obstruction at the skin level will respond, at least temporarily, to the removal of the constricting band.

(c) Prolapse

Prolapse of the bud, as with recession, may be fixed or sliding. It is associated with emotional difficulties because the prolapsed stoma is ugly, and mechanical problems arise because the protruding bowel pushes the ileostomy appliance away from the abdominal wall, thus producing leakage followed by excoriation.

Treatment. A fixed prolapse can easily be treated by amputation. The mucocutaneous junction is dissected free and the two layers of bowel separated. The latter manoeuvre is simple because the layers are usually bound together by flimsy adhesions. Once separated, sufficient length of bowel is removed to restore the bud to a reasonable size.

If the prolapse is sliding, a major intra-abdominal procedure is necessary in order to refix the mesentery and the bowel to the abdominal wall.

(d) Fistula

This is a wholly avoidable complication usually caused through wearing an ill-fitting ileostomy ring or one that has ridden across the abdominal wall and ulcerated through the wall of the bowel. All fistulae form at skin level (Fig. 2.21) and once they have formed there is skin excoriation followed by difficulties in controlling the effluent. Local treatment is useless, and an intra-abdominal reconstruction of the ileostomy is required.

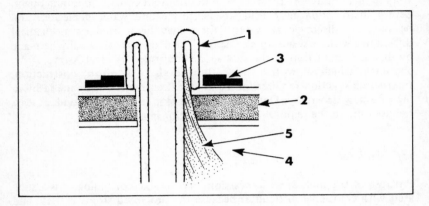

Fig 2.21   Formal ileostomy as described by Brooke
1. Ileostomy bud   2. Abdominal parietes   3. Adhesive ring   4. Lateral space
5. Mesentery of small bowel

(e) Herniation

This is a relatively rare complication which could demand, if difficulty arose with the ileostomy apparatus, resiting the ileostomy on the opposite side of the abdomen and closure of the defect.

(f) Skin excoriation

Any mismanagement or disturbance, however temporary, of an ileostomy may lead to contamination of the surrounding skin followed by excoriation. This is generally ameliorated by using Karaya gum powder (Pulv. Sterculis B.P.C), which functions as an adhesive even in the presence of skin ulceration, thus protecting the involved skin. The powder may be applied by dusting it over the skin around the ileostomy, adding water, and then following with more powder, the process being repeated several times until a thick glue-like layer has been produced. An alternative dressing is to use Squibb's Stomahesive, which has the appearance of a wafer of thin toffee. A hole is cut in the wafer to the exact dimensions of the ileostomy, the wafer is then applied to the excoriated abdominal wall, after which the flange is applied. This is a neater, but more costly way of achieving healing.

The continent ileostomy

Because the formal ileostomy as perfected by Turnbull of America and Brooke of England remains incontinent throughout its existence it must inevitably mean that some form of apparatus must be continuously worn, and although improvement in the overall design and in the quality of adhesive have improved dramatically a significant number of patients still complain of skin problems.

It was to avoid this particular deficiency of the classic ileostomy that Koch in 1969, proposed an entirely new procedure in which the terminal ileum is converted into a reservoir and, finally, after many modifications of the original technique, a nipple valve was constructed which passed from the reservoir to the skin surface (Figs 2.22, 2.23). Should all go well this technique produces total continence and so the reservoir must be intermittently emptied by means of a catheter inserted through the stoma which is flush with the skin and into the reservoir. The catheter must be carried at all times since the perfect operation is designed to produce total obstruction. Initially, the reservoir, which is formed by folding the terminal 45 to 50 cm of ileum, holds only 100 to 200 ml of ileal contents, but as time passes its capacity normally increases until it is capable of holding between 500 to 1000 ml. The critical procedure is the formation of the nipple valve since if this fails to operate the reservoir is incontinent and the patient is in fact worse off than with a formal ileostomy because the stoma is normally sutured flush with the skin, making the control

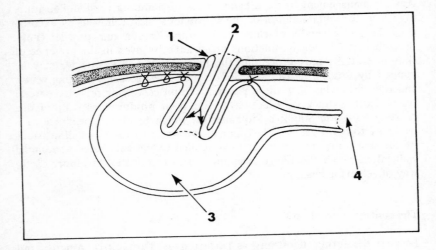

Fig 2.22   Saggital section through Koch's continent ileostomy
1. Ileal mucosa sutured directly to skin   2. Interssuscepted ileum producing the 'nipple valve'   3. Reservoir formed from terminal 40 cm of ileum   4. Terminal ileum entering reservoir

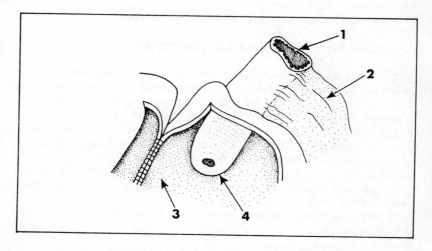

Fig. 2.23   Ileostomy: reservoir opened to show projection of nipple valve
1. Cut end of ileum to be brought to the surface   2. Mesentery   3. Internal aspect of
reservoir   4. Nipple valve projecting into reservoir

of any discharge virtually impossible. The final appearance of the valve, which is formed by intussuscepting the terminal ileum into the reservoir, is shown in Figs. 2.22 and 2.23.

Despite the theoretical advantages this type of ileostomy possesses over the traditional and now well-tried procedure, many surgeons remain critical of its use since a number of serious complications have been described. These include—

(a) necrosis of the reservoir,
(b) extrusion of the valve with resulting incontinence,
(c) volvulus of the reservoir,
(d) perforation of the reservoir during catheterisation.

Should necrosis of the reservoir come about from any cause and the pouch has to be resected it means that the terminal 50 cm of ileum will be lost. This may be followed by serious absorptive difficulties making the ileostomy discharge more fluid and, therefore, more difficult to control. It has been clearly shown that the excision of 60 cm of the terminal ileum produces an outflow of over 1 litre in the majority of patients, whereas when the resection is limited to less than 10 cm the outflow is less than 0.5 litre. Such a volume with its attendant loss of sodium is dangerous and requires the continuous administration of codeine phosphate or Lomotil for its control.

It cannot be too strongly stressed that this operation is not one that should be attempted by a surgeon who is called upon to perform an ileostomy at infrequent intervals.

2.14 THE USE OF ULTRASONOGRAPHY IN SURGICAL DIAGNOSIS

PRINCIPLES

Ultrasound is energy in the form of mechanical vibration in which the vibration has a frequency in excess of that to which the human ear is sensitive, i.e. 20 to 20 000 MHz. The operating range of the majority of ultrasonic frequencies is between 0.5 and 20 MHz. Ultrasonic energy travels in the form of a wave which is usually longitudinal and the particles of the transmitting material vibrate backwards and forwards.

Ultrasound, used for diagnostic purposes is generated and detected by the piezoelectric effect, both processes involving conversion between electrical and mechanical energies. This effect was first discovered in 1880 by J and P Curie who noted that the compression of certain crystalline materials produced an electric discharge so long as the crystal had been cut in planes parallel to those natural to the crystal. Piezoelectric materials are called transducers, because they provide a coupling between electrical and mechanical energies. The electric charges bound within the ionic lattice of the material are arranged in such a way that they can react with an applied electric field to produce a mechanical effect and vice versa.

Many naturally occurring crystals are piezoelectric, e.g. quartz, but the most commonly used material for the making of ultrasonic diagnostic equipment is the synthetic ceramic lead zirconate titanate, which belongs to a group of materials known as the ferroelectrics.

The narrow ultrasonic beam required for diagnostic purposes is most commonly generated by a disc of peizoelectric material electrically excited by means of two electrodes, one on each parallel surface. When an alternating voltage is applied between the electrodes, the piezoelectric effect causes a synchronous variation in the thickness of the transducer. The movements of the surfaces of the transducer then radiate energy into the media which are adjacent to them, the proportion depending upon the density of the media and the velocity of the waves.

BASIS OF DIAGNOSTIC CAPABILITY

With few exceptions a diagnosis using ultrasound depends upon the fact that ultrasonic waves are reflected from naturally occurring boundaries between different tissues within the body, a fraction of the energy being reflected if there is impedance at such a boundary. Energy that is not reflected travels onwards, although the depth to which it can penetrate is limited by the attenuation of the wave as it passes through the tissues.

Since ultrasound is almost completely reflected at boundaries between air and solids the application of this technique is seriously restricted. It is for this reason, too, that air must be excluded, by means of a liquid coupling medium, from the point of contact between the transducer and the patient. In contrast, the propagation velocity and the attentuation of ultrasound is much greater in bones than in soft tissues, hence examination of bones by this technique is unsatisfactory.

Advantages and disadvantages of ultrasonography

The advantages of ultrasonography are:
(*a*)   It is a non-invasive technique which causes, at diagnostic levels, no overt tissue damage such as may potentially follow radiology or other electromagnetic scanning techniques. It is because of this that it can be safely used in obstetric practice. (*b*) It requires minimal patient co-operation. A study normally takes only 10 to 30 minutes and has the advantage of being completely painless.

The disadvantages are that gas, trabeculated bone, and barium sulphate reflect ultrasonic waves, hence, there is no penetration. Thus, gas-containing structures such as the gastrointestinal and respiratory tracts cannot be adequately visualised by this technique nor can abnormalities in bone be detected.

METHOD OF USE

There are three chief ways in which ultrasound can be used: the pulse-echo method, the B-scan, and the Doppler method.

(a) Pulse-echo method

When an ultrasonic pulse strikes the boundary between two media of different impedance, the delay that transpires between the transmission of the pulse and the reception of its echo depends upon the velocity of the impulse and the length of the track to and from the reflecting surface. The velocity is relatively constant, a transit of 10 mm occurring in 6.7 μs.

In this type of scan, also known as the A-scan, the information received from the reflected sound waves is displayed on a cathode-ray tube and appears as a series of deflections, the number of which depends upon the number of interfaces through which the waves have travelled. The usefulness of this particular method is somewhat limited by the multiple reflections or reverberations the ultrasonic pulse may undergo during its propagation. This is because, once the reflected wave has returned to the face of the probe it is re-reflected back into the medium into which it was initially propagated. This reflected pulse then behaves as if it were a second pulse and, although it is of smaller amplitude than the first, a series of reverberation artefacts are produced.

(b) B-scan

The information obtained by the pulse-echo method, comprising a combination of data relating to range and amplitude, can also be displayed on a brightness-modulated time-base in such a way that the brightness increases with the echo-amplitude; hence, by mounting the ultrasonic probe on a mechanical scanner that allows movement in two directions a tomograph may be obtained. The advantage of the so-called grey-scale display, introduced in 1972, in which the echoes back scattered from the tissue interfaces may be displayed in as many as 12 shades between white and black, is its ability to detect subtle changes from within organs and structures.

This is achieved by selective amplification of the low level echoes that originate from the interfaces within soft tissues. The 'shade' obtained is dependent upon the primary tissue state, so that supportive elements within tissues such as collagen and elastin may be 'visualised'. Thus, a cirrhotic liver can be distinguished from a normal liver because the latter is replaced by fibrous tissue.

(c) Ultrasonic Doppler methods

These are now widely used for the study of moving structures. The Doppler shift in frequency of a continuous wave ultrasonic beam reflected from a moving structure can be used to provide information about the velocity of the structure, e.g. blood, which may be detected either by ear or by instrumentation. In obstetrics and cardiology the frequency generally used is between 2 and 3 MHz but in blood flow studies it may be as high as 10 MHz.

APPLICATION TO DIAGNOSTIC PROBLEMS

Hepatobiliary system

The liver

In practice the liver is scanned by the use of the 'acoustic window' (Fig. 2.24) which lies between the lung above and the air-conditioning colon below. The patient inspires deeply and the transducer is angled under the right costal margin after a suitable coupling agent such as mineral oil has been applied to the skin. The scans are made in a series of parasagittal planes. A section taken 20 mm to the left of the midline shows the aorta posteriorly and the left lobe of the liver anteriorly; 20 mm to the right of the midline the lumen of the inferior vena cava can be recognised with the portal vein lying somewhat anteriorly as it ascends towards the hilum of the liver. The sensitivity of the method is such that the increased diameter of the portal vein, which occurs in cirrhosis, can easily be recognised.

Discrete hepatic lesions

The common discrete liver abnormalities for the detection of which ultrasonography may be usefully employed include metastatic disease, abscess formation, cystic disease, and primary hepatomas.

(*a*) In the majority of patients suffering from *hepatic metastases* there are multiple areas which return echoes of slightly lower amplitude than the normal intervening liver tissue. Hepatic lymphomas, being highly homogeneous, produce such low echo levels that they may even simulate abscess cavities.

(*b*) *Abscesses* within the liver or subphrenic abscesses lying between the diaphragm and upper surface of the right lobe produce areas that return abnormally low level echoes, the amplitude depending upon the fluidity of the abscess contents.

(*c*) *Cysts* of the liver (Fig. 2.25) may be congenital or acquired. Congenital benign cysts appear as well-defined structures with smooth walls, and from within the cyst there is a total absence of echoes, due to the non-reflective nature of the homogeneous fluid within the cyst. Posterior to

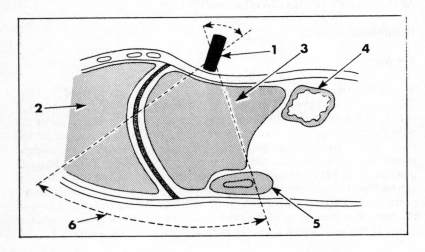

Fig. 2.24   The acoustic window of the liver
1. Transducer   2. Lung   3. Liver   4. Colon   5. Kidney   6. Limits of sector scan

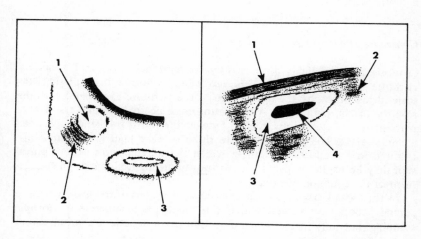

Left

Fig 2.25   Simple cyst of the liver (*see* page 173)
1. Cyst   2. Enhanced echoes from area posterior to cyst   3. Kidney

Right

Fig 2.26   Posterior longitudinal scan kidney approximately 70 mm to the right of the midline
1. Posterior abdominal wall   2. Perinephric fat   3. Renal parenchyma   4. Renal pelvis and calyces

the site of the cyst there is commonly an increase in the returning echoes. This confirms the fluid content of the lesion and occurs because more sound has reached and therefore, has been reflected from the tissues behind the cyst.

(d) *Primary hepatomas* produce homogenous irregular areas with poorly defined borders and occasional internal echoes, which, if present, indicate necrotic degeneration.

Generalised liver disease

Cirrhosis can be reliably diagnosed by conventional ultrasound because a cirrhotic liver returns higher echo levels than a normal organ. Using grey scale ultrasonography the appearance of the cirrhotic liver varies with the severity of the pathology. Attentuation may be so high that the deeper parts of the liver are only reached by examination at frequencies between 1 and 2 HMz. The appearances are those of very high level echoes distributed in a scattered pattern in which the dilated and tortuous portal vein may be readily apparent, its tortuosity distinguishing it from enlargement of the common bile duct.

In the overall diagnosis of space-occupying lesions of the liver substance several papers have suggested that this technique is superior to isotopic scanning, not only in the actual detection of an hepatic lesion but also in determining its nature.

Biliary tract

This investigation is useful for—

1 The detection of a distended gall-bladder, seen particularly well on a paramedian liver scan. This, of course, may be caused by a carcinoma of the common bile duct, the ampulla of Vater, or the head of the pancreas and, occasionally, a mucocele of the gall-bladder.

2 The diagnosis of gall-stones. These can be visualised even when they are not radio-opaque. A marked shadowing effect may be seen beyond the stone due to the severe attenuation of the beam during its passage through the stone or stones.

3 The recognition of a dilated common bile duct. This abnormality is particularly well seen in paramedian sections taken 20 mm to the right of the midline. Should the investigator be able to trace the duct inferiorly the site of obstruction may be identified, and if the ducts are traced proximally the intrahepatic ducts, if sufficiently dilated, can also be recognised.

4 To distinguish between extra and intrahepatic causes of jaundice.

In one recently reported series an accurate diagnosis of extrahepatic obstruction was made in 64 out of 66 patients. The distinction between these two causes of jaundice rests upon the differing dimensions of the biliary canaliculi, hepatic ducts, and common bile duct. Since the gall-bladder may not communicate with the remainder of the biliary tree any conclusions based on its size may be spurious.

The advantages of ultrasonic scanning in the diagnosis of hepatobiliary disease are—

(a)   its non-invasive nature;
(b)   because conventional oral and intravenous cholangiograms are unlikely to be successful in the presence of clinical jaundice;
(c)   because percutaneous cholangiography, even when performed using a Chiba needle, and endoscopic retrograde cholangiopancreatography are both not without risk, are considerably more time consuming, and require the use of more manpower and technology.

The Pancreas

Pancreatic disease

Examination of the distal part of the body and tail of the pancreas are difficult because they lie behind the stomach and transverse colon, but the head and body can be visualised by making use of the acoustic window of the liver. Normal pancreatic tissue produces a cobblestone mosaic with differing depth of echo attentuation.

Pancreatic tumours

Pancreatic tumours appear as irregular masses but must be some 3 to 4 cm in diameter before they can be distinguished from the normal surrounding pancreatic tissue.

Pancreatitis

Acute pancreatitis, even an acute or chronic attack, can be diagnosed by ultrasonography because the development of oedema increases the permeability of the organ to sound, its outlines therefore becoming easier to detect. The inflamed pancreas shows as a transonic arc-shaped plate.

Complications of pancreatitis

Ultrasonography is of greatest value, however, in the diagnosis of pancreatic pseudocysts, a relatively common complication of acute pancreatitis. Pancreatic cysts appear as rounded echo-free masses lying adjacent to the body or tail of the pancreas. If this diagnosis is suspected the stomach must be completely empty before examination is begun, otherwise confusion may arise since a dilated fluid-filled stomach can produce a similar picture.

Urogenital tract

The kidneys, lying in the retroperitoneal tissues are 'covered' anteriorly by gas-filled loops of bowel; in consequence, direct 'vision' through the peritoneal cavity is difficult. However, by using the acoustic window provided by the liver the right kidney may be scanned and sometimes the left may also be seen. Because of these technical difficulties the kidneys are commonly scanned in the prone position, when a series of longitudinal scans can be made parallel to the spine at intervals of 5 to 10 mm, usually beginning 60 mm from the midline as this passes through the kidney.

It is usually considered that ultrasound examination should be preceded by intravenous pyelography, which will itself give a fairly accurate picture of many renal conditions. However, a pyelographic distinction between cyst and tumour may be difficult to make since both may produce enlargement of the renal outline and both may produce the deformity of the pelvi-calcyceal system known as the 'spider calyx'.

A longitudinal scan of a normal kidney shows the readily recognisable oval, smooth outline of the kidney, with the calices, pelvis and blood vessels forming a central group of high amplitude echoes (Fig. 2.26). When the scan passes lateral to the calices no central echo will be found. In transverse scans the normal kidney is obviously oval or rounded in shape, and the calices produce a group of echoes which are nearly central in position when the scan passes through one of the renal poles, or is medially placed if the scan goes through the renal pelvis. Above or below the calices the central echo is absent and the ureters are unidentifiable unless they are dilated.

Von Grawitz or renal cell carinoma (Fig. 2.27)

A renal tumour normally indents, displaces, or destroys a part of the kidney and caliceal system which results in the organ losing its regular outline and being replaced by a mass which, because of its heterogenous nature produces multiple random echoes, the necrotic parts of the neoplasm having a very low echogenicity in comparison with the solid areas.

These findings are in direct contra-distinction to a renal cyst which also commonly deforms the kidney. However, in contra-distinction to a tumour, which may produce an irregular outline, a cyst is usually well defined. In addition, because of the homogeneous nature of a cyst's contents no echoes arise from within the cyst on the A or B scan because the ultrasound is only slightly attenuated by the fluid in the cyst. There is also an area of relatively higher intensity echoes deep to the cyst (Fig. 2.28).

The various papers published on the use of ultrasound for the diagnosis of renal masses suggest that the method is very reliable.

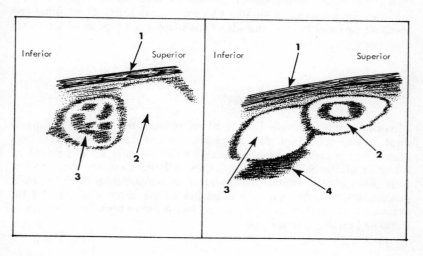

Left

Fig 2.27   Renal carcinoma
1. Posterior abdominal wall   2. Kidney   3. Tumour

Right

Fig 2.28   Renal cyst
1. Posterior abdominal wall   2. Kidney   3. Cyst   4. Enhancement echoes posterior to the cyst

Hydronephrosis

The diagnosis of hydronephrosis by ultrasonic methods depends on the degree of pelvic dilatation which, in turn, produces separation of the central echoes. This causes a ring of echoes in a longitudinal scan, and in advanced cases, particularly those in which there is a large element of extra renal hydronephrosis, the dilated pelvis can be identified as a transonic mass lying medial to the kidney. Should the cause be an impacted stone this may be apparent as an area of dense echogenicity in an otherwise anechoic area and beyond the site of the stone will be the usual ultrasonic shadowing.

Miscellaneous urological conditions

Ultrasonography has also been used to measure the residual volume of urine in patients complaining of prostatism, but the method is relatively inaccurate. It can also be used to assess the presence or absence of infiltration of the bladder wall in patients suffering from bladder tumours. Infiltration of the bladder wall produces an increase in its thickness and a general lack of definition. The reliability of the latter is increased if the examination is performed when the bladder is full or urine and the tumour is situated on its posterior wall.

The Brain

The range of structures that lie in the cerebral median sagittal plane from the surface of the scalp can be measured by an ultrasonic pulse-echo technique—'midline echoencephalography'. A significant difference in the ranges measured from either side of the head suggests that the cerebral mid-line structures have been displaced although the precise nature of the lesion responsible for such displacement may not be determined. A midline 'shift' following an acute injury is most commonly caused by an intracranial haemorrhage situated in an extra or subdural intracerebral position.

In a patient suffering a head injury which is followed by severe generalised cerebral oedema, the interhemispheric fissure tends to be obliterated as the interfaces on either side of it are pressed together. The result is that the echogenicity of this interface is reduced and it may not be so easily identified. It is for this reason that in the performance of mid-line echoencephalography the investigator must be aware of the full clinical history and the potential underlying pathology.

In chronic conditions the displacement may be the result of a brain tumour or, alternatively, the midline may be drawn to the affected side by an atrophic lesion such as an old clot or cerebral infarct.

However, so far as the brain is concerned this investigation has now been replaced in those hospitals in which the apparatus is available, by computer-assisted axial tomography which, like ultrasonography, is a non-invasive technique.

The Vascular system

(a) *Anatomical disease.* The normal size and any alteration in shape in the form of an abdominal aortic aneurysm can be readily detected by longitudinal scanning of the abdominal wall from the level of the xiphoid to the symphysis. It is also extremely easy to recognise the presence of intra-anaeurysmal thrombosis.

(b) *Physiological changes produced by anatomical disease.* The blood flow in a peripheral artery may be measured by adopting the Doppler principle. If a Doppler flow-detector is traced along the course of an artery, two component sounds are heard superimposed on a continuous low-frequency signal. The first corresponding to systole, is high pitched, and the second, corresponding to diastole, is low pitched.

It is, however, now possible to measure velocity-time wave forms by making recordings simultaneously at separate sites on the limb, usually between the common femoral and the popliteal arteries or the popliteal and the posterior tibial artery behind the medial malleolus of the ankle. Blood pressure measurements which can be made by the Doppler technique can also be used to evaluate the run-off vessels in the arterial system of a limb by measuring the cuff occlusion pressure at several segments along the limb.

In a similar fashion continuous wave Doppler can provide a rapid and reliable indication of the patency of the vascular supply to a transplanted kidney, a diminishing flow velocity warning that rejection is imminent.

2.15 USES OF RADIOACTIVE ISOTOPES IN SURGERY

Isotopes are elements that contain the same number of protons but a different number of neutrons within the nucleus, the latter differentiating them from the normal element. Difference in the number of neutrons produces an element that is indistinguishable chemically but one which has a nucleus that is unstable and, therefore, liable to undergo spontaneous disintegration, resulting in the release of alpha, beta, or gamma particles.

Detection of Emission

Alpha, beta or gamma particles can be detected by a variety of different methods, e.g. photographic film, ionisation detectors, geiger counters, or scintillation detectors. Scintillation detectors, which are in common use, convert irradiation into photons of visible or ultraviolet light by interaction with crystals such as sodium iodide.

SURGICAL APPLICATIONS OF ISOTOPES

Isotope studies have been applied to the solution of surgical problems in four ways—

1 for tumour detection;
2 for the visual recording of the progress of a disease;
3 as a test of organ function;
4 as therapeutic agents.

Tumour detection in bone

A common example of the use of isotopes for tumour detection is their application to detect bone metastases, particularly in patients suffering from carcinoma of the breast. Isotope surveys of the skeleton are considerably more sensitive than plain X-rays.

Bone scanning is performed by administering a bone-seeking nuclide, among which are ^{18}F, ^{47}Ca, ^{87}Sr and ^{85}Sr. ^{18}F is seldom used because it is cyclotron produced and has a half-life of only 168 minutes; because of this the patient must live near or be brought to the source of production. A more commonly used isotope is ^{87m}Sr which has a lower gamma output than other isotopes.

Factors governing the uptake of the isotope

The uptake of a bone-seeking nuclide is governed by three major factors—

1 The rate of substitution of the isotope used for stable calcium and hydroxyl ions; this reaction probably occurs in amorphous calcium phosphate which is a precursor of hydroxyappatite.
2 Bone blood flow, which influences the delivery of an isotope into areas of activity.
3 Hormonal influences, because these govern the quantitative aspects of mineralisation.

^{85}Sr can be detected on a bone scan when its local concentration has reached approximately three times the normal value. Any reactive process within the bone that results in either a translucency or increased density on the plain radiograph always produces an abnormal scan.

One of the chief advantages of isotope scanning is that abnormalities in the calcium content of a bone can be detected by this means much sooner than by a plain X-ray, often by several months, because changes in the latter occur only after the calcium content has fallen by 30 to 50 per cent.

However, the changes observed on a bone scan are wholly non-specific and such an examination should always be preceded by a careful history, physical examination, and the performance of those biochemical tests which normally indicate bone disease, if abnormal. These tests include measurement of the serum calcium and urinary calcium excretion, the alkaline phosphatase, and the urinary creatinine/hydroxyproline ratio.

Isotopic surveys of the skeleton may be used by the surgeon in one of two ways: for screening apparently well women, or for the confirmation of already suspected bone lesions.

In women suffering from carcinoma of the breast, numerous surveys have shown that a relatively large proportion of women with apparently curable cancer have 'hot spots' in the skeleton. Time is required, however, to assess the true significance of these findings.

In patients suffering from carcinoma of the bladder a skeletal survey is especially indicated before total cystectomy, because the presence of asymptomatic bony secondaries should make the surgeon hesitate before performing such a major procedure.

Diagnostically, a skeletal scan is appropriate when a bony lesion is suspected but remains unconfirmed on plain radiographs, possibly because of overlying soft tissue shadows. A scan nearly always shows a greater degree of bone change than is suspected from the radiographic appearance of the lesion.

Negative bone scan

A scan may sometimes be negative even in the presence of a bony lesion if there is rapid bone destruction without any associated reactive osteogenesis. Conversely, stable secondaries, which sometimes occur in thyroid cancer, may also produce little if any observable changes.

Brain Scans

Brain scanning can now be effectively used for—

(a)   the diagnosis of intracranial space-occupying lesions;
(b)   the estimation of cerebral blood flow.

The following isotopes have been used ^{99m}Tc, ^{197}Hg-chlormerodin and ^{113m} indium chelate. Iodinated macroaggregated albumin has also been used but this is potentially dangerous because of the particle size which is such that it may block the cerebral capillaries.

(a) Tumour diagnosis

Three factors largely determine whether a tumour can be identified by scanning techniques—

1 the differential uptake pattern;
2 the location of the tumour;
3 the size of the tumour.

Peripheral tumours lying within normal brain tissue are more easily distinguished from normal brain tissue than are central tumours such as pinealomas, and the vascular pattern at the base of the skull frequently makes tumours in this area difficult to locate. In terms of pathology, meningiomas, glioblastomas and metastatic lesions are more easily located than the less vascular astrocytomas.

(b) Estimation of cerebral blood flow

This investigation is of particular interest to the surgeon when considering the clinical significance of carotid artery stenosis.

Liver Scans

Colloidal ^{198}Au, aggregated human ^{131}I-albumin, or a sulphated colloid labelled with technetium ^{99}mTc are most frequently used for hepatic scanning. All are taken up within 10 to 15 minutes by the reticuloendo-thelial cells of the liver. ^{131}I-albumin results in the least hepatic irradiation because it is rapidly destroyed and eliminated in the urine. Other materials, taken up by the liver cells themselves, include ^{131}I labelled Rose-Bengal and ^{131}I labelled PVP. An area of high radioactivity is produced when functioning hepatic tissue takes up radioactive substances.

Uses of Liver Scan

1 Detection of subphrenic abscess

In this condition the liver may be displaced downwards by the developing abscess. In such a patient if the liver scan is superimposed upon the plain radiograph the space between the upper surface of the liver and the diaphragm is demonstrated. Alternatively, if a combined lung and liver scan are performed the space between the two viscera caused by the presence of an abscess will be demonstrated. Drainage and cure of the abscess leads to closer apposition of the two scans.

Intrahepatic defects as small as 20 mm in diameter can now be detected but a scan alone will not differentiate between an abscess, a cyst, or a neoplasm. Occasionally, a hepatoma may, however, because of its cellular composition, show as an area of increased radioactivity, the hot liver nodule.

Lung Scanning

The common agents used for lung scanning are ^{131}I labelled macro-aggregated albumin, or ^{99}mTc labelled albumin. Before administration of ^{131}I labelled preparations sodium iodide should be administered to minimise accumulation of the isotope in the thyroid. The posture of the patient is important because the pulmonary circulation is a low-pressure system. In the erect position, the lung fields are increasingly dense from the apices to the bases. To achieve an even distribution of the isotope through the lung fields it should be injected slowly with the patient in either the supine or the erect position.

Four standard projections of the perfused lung are normally taken; the posterior, anterior, and right and left lateral. The posterior view is the most important projection because it encompasses the greatest volume of lung. In the lateral views the opposite lung makes approximately a 30 per cent contribution to the image of the lung being scanned.

Pulmonary embolus

A major indication for lung scanning is a suspected pulmonary embolus. This condition is sometimes notoriously silent because more than 50 per cent of the pulmonary arteriolar bed must be occluded before there is a significant alteration in cardiopulmonary haemodynamics.

This investigation is unnecessary when the diagnosis is clinically obvious or when simpler investigations such as a plain radiograph of the chest will suffice. The scan is positive when areas of regional ischaemia of lobar or segmental distribution can be seen. Additional information, if necessary, could be obtained by pulmonary angiography but this is seldom required.

Serial scans have shown that an embolus can be cleared with remarkable rapidity in an individual with previously healthy lungs. However, in congestive heart failure, or when old emboli reach the lung, clearing is slower.

Miscellaneous pulmonary conditions

A large number of different types of pulmonary and pleural masses can be demonstrated by scanning techniques. As in other areas, however, the scan, while demonstrating the defect in the lung fields, gives little or no help in the precise diagnosis.

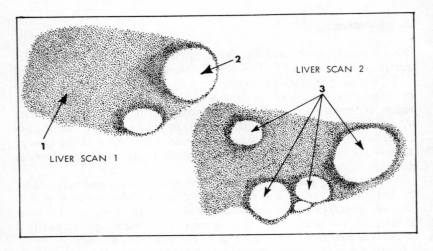

Fig 2.29 Serial liver scan showing progressive development of defects from secondary deposits arising from a carcinoma of the colon
1. Liver substance   2. Defect   3. Multiple defects seen several months later

Pancreatic scanning

The principles of pancreatic scanning are as follows: first, the pancreas may be emptied of its pre-existing enzymes by an injection of secretin and pancreazymin; secondly, the liver is outlined with colloidal ^{198}Au, after which a dose of selenium tagged methionine is given. ^{75}Se has a half-life of 128 days; it is incorporated into the methionine molecule in place of sulphur, producing a gamma-emitting amino acid. The uptake of seleno-methionine is related to the level of enzyme synthesis, and in the first hour after administration about 7 per cent is localised in the pancreas, the maximum uptake being within 30 minutes. In a normal scan, the neck, body, and tail assume either a straight or sigmoid configuration in relation to the head.

This investigation is not often used because there are other, in general terms, more effective investigations. These include retrograde cannulation of the pancreatic duct via the Ampulla of Vater in order to perform a retrograde pancreatogram, the use of ultrasound and, lastly, pancreatic arteriography.

Value of a Pancreatic Scan

The diagnostic accuracy of a pancreatic scan in patients who are clinically suspected of pancreatic disease is of the order of 70 per cent. False negatives are relatively uncommon but false positives tend to detract from the value of this investigation. Carcinoma of the body and tail may produce circumscribed areas of diminished uptake and associated distortion of the surrounding normal tissues.

The appearance of the scan is variable in the presence of a pancreatic pseudocyst. If the cyst communicates with a major pancreatic duct, due to a high concentration of enzymes, there may be an area of increased activity but this is a comparatively rare finding.

Renal Scanning

Techniques

^{131}I-iodohippurate, which is excreted into the renal tubules by a combination of glomerular filtration and tubular secretion, is commonly used. It is almost completely extracted from the blood with each passage through the kidneys (99 per cent) and since 25 per cent of the cardiac output is channelled through the kidneys within a period of 2½ to 5 minutes all the rapidly accumulating radiohippuran is within view of a renal detector.

Uses

Isotope techniques allow a semi-quantitative measurement of renal blood flow, renal function, and the anatomical size and shape of the kidneys. The type of clinical problem in which isotope techniques may, therefore, be helpful are—

1 the determination of unilateral alterations in renal function caused, for example, by renal artery stenosis;
2 the presence of obstructive uropathy;
3 the diagnosis of a space-occupying lesion.

Although applicable to all these problems, alternative methods of investigation exist.

Normal renogram (Fig. 2.30)

The rate at which the isotope appears in the kidney and collecting system is dependent on two major factors—

(*a*) the amount of blood flowing through the kidney,
(*b*) the function of the tubule cells.

The normal renogram is composed of three slopes. An initial slope of negligible duration which rises almost vertically; an intermediate slope lasting for some 3.5 minutes, which is approximately 70° to the horizontal; and a third slope equivalent in angle but in the reverse direction, which lasts for several minutes.

When renal function is decreased or the blood flow diminished, the second slope becomes flatter, and with ever-decreasing function finally disappears. When the kidney is obstructed the third phase may be eliminated as the excreted isotope cannot drain down the ureter.

To determine the anatomical size and shape of the kidneys a rectilinear scanning device is normally used, giving ^{197}Hg – chlormerodin some two hours before beginning the scan. This compound is temporarily bound in the renal tubules, and therefore, very little is excreted in the urine for approximately two hours. This method delineates filling defects or areas of infarction.

Thyroid Scanning and Function

See Section 2.1 and Section 3.2 Tutorials in Surgery I.

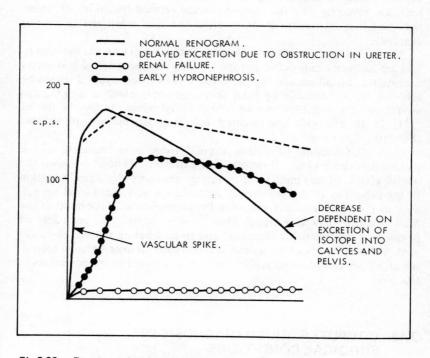

Fig 2.30   Renogram showing normal and abnormal patterns

If a thyroid cancer, particularly a metastatic thyroid cancer, can take up
^{131}I, this may form a useful method of treatment. It implies some degree
of differentiation of the tumour for the anaplastic carcinomas cannot be
treated by this method due to a lack of uptake.

The majority of surgeons would accept that the primary treatment of
thyroid cancer is surgical, especially when the cancer is confined to the
neck, i.e. involving only the thyroid and the cervical lymph nodes, unless
the condition is inoperable as is often the case when the tumour is
anaplastic.

A major problem has always been to stimulate extracervical deposits to
take up sufficient radioactive isotope for their destruction, and in order to
accomplish this all normal thyroid tissue must be destroyed. This can be
achieved either surgically by total thyroidectomy, which carries the disadvantage of a high incidence of hypoparathyroidism, or by the use of
^{131}I; 75 to 150 mCi administered following an injection of thyroid
stimulating hormone.

Only after ablation of normal thyroid tissue does treatment of the
metastatic disease begin. However, it is extremely difficult to assess the
overall effects of this method of treatment because of biological variation
in the behaviour of thyroid cancer. Both the age and histological appearance of the tumour greatly influence the survival time. McDermott of the
Massachusetts General Hospital found, for example, that regardless of
histological type, patients diagnosed and treated before the age of 40 did
well, with a mortality of 8 per cent, whereas patients over 40 had a mortality of 58 per cent. Similar results have been reported by other workers in
this field.

2.16 COMPUTER-AIDED DIAGNOSIS IN SURGICAL CONDITIONS

In 1969, Professor Card of the University of Glasgow posed the question,
can the computer solve any clinical problems and, if so, what fraction?
He pointed out that the ultimate object of medicine in its broadest sense
is to improve the quality of life and its quantity in as many people as
possible. The author would demur somewhat, considering that subjectively
and objectively, quality is of much greater importance than quantity.

Traditional diagnostic method

However, before ill-health can be treated a diagnosis is required and the
number of diagnoses is increasing rapidly as our knowledge of the pathological and physiological changes accompanying a particular illness expand.

Essentially, a clinical diagnosis is made by correlating the data derived from the patient by interrogation, clinical examination and, finally, the investigation of the patient.

Traditionally the patient is interrogated by his/her doctor, physician, or surgeon. This has the definite advantage of helping to establish and cement a doctor/patient relationship, and the somewhat less precise advantage that the doctor supposedly knows the most pertinent questions to ask. A less orthodox method of interrogation is to use a medical assistant who starts with no medical knowledge, and, therefore, theoretically with no bias towards a particular diagnosis, but who is trained to interrogate patients suffering from a selected group of diseases. Even less orthodox would be history-taking by computer.

Computer interrogation

This method involves the use of a visual display unit with a specially designed keyboard on which to record the responses. This method was first used in the United States in the early sixties by Slack for interrogating patients suffering from various allergies and has recently been used in the United Kingdom.

In the system used in the UK, apart from the obvious *Yes, No, Don't understand* responses, qualified answers such as *commonly, probably,* and *possibly* were also built into the system, together with a decision algorithm allocating patients to a three or seven button response according to age and verbal intelligence. Analysis of the results of such methods of interrogation showed that the attitude of any particular patient was influenced by age, sex, and occupation. Males under 30 years of age engaged in manual work appeared to be more impressed, and accepted computerised interrogation more easily and favourably than professional and older groups of patients.

The clinical history having been recorded, examination and, if necessary, investigation of the patient naturally follows. The weighing of the total evidence and the making of a judgement involves the clinician in assessing how likely it is that the various features under consideration occur in a particular disease. Such an assessment is made in the light of his/her own past experience and in that of others, taking into account the incidence of the particular features of what he/she considers the most likely disease. Diagnosis is often accomplished without any difficulty but errors may sometimes occur since even experienced observers may in their assessment find it difficult to decide what relative importance should be attached to different data. However, the majority of clinicians with increasing experience come to recognise patterns of symptoms and signs and almost certainly subconsciously assess the probability of their occurrence in different diseases.

Since this is the method by which the human mind works it is not impossible to envisage a system in which the correct diagnosis might be calculated for a particular patient by a formal application of the probability theory. This method involves the prior collection of a considerable mass of clinical data, which must be collected in a relatively formalised manner and stored in a computer as a data base. The formation of the latter is a long and tedious process and has so far been applied to few clinical problems, among which are the differential diagnosis of acute abdominal pain, dyspepsia, and jaundice.

Construction of data base

A data base necessary for the diagnosis of the different causes of acute abdominal pain was constructed by deDombal and his colleages in 1971 by interrogating and examining a series of 600 patients suffering from acute abdominal distress. The diseases with which this group were particularly concerned were acute appendicitis, diverticulitis, perforated peptic ulceration, cholecystitis, small bowel obstruction, pancreatitis and non-specific abdominal pain. A total of 42 clinical attributes were assessed for each of the 600 patients so that the database when completed consisted of about 25,000 items of clinical information. A mass of clinical data of this magnitude allows separate consideration of each of the 42 attributes and allows definition of those features that are judged the most useful in discriminating between the various diseases.

Bayesian analysis

The computer diagnosis is made by an entry, i.e. the details of the history and clinical examination of the, as yet, undiagnosed patient, into the computer which then performs a Bayesian analysis based on the previously entered data. Although widely known for some time the application of Bayes's theorem to statistical analysis has been extremely limited by the controversy that exists over the necessary assignment of the 'prior probabilities', but although this controversy remains, increasing use of the method is being made.

Essentially, the theorem is as follows. Suppose we have a set of possible alternative disease diagnoses $D_1, D_2, D_3 \ldots D_n$ for a given patient A, one of which will be 'nothing wrong' and of which one and only one will be correct. Before a given medical examination E, suppose the associated respective probabilities, known as the prior probabilities are $p_1, p_2, p_3 \ldots p_n$, then $p_1 + p_2 + p_3 + p_n = 1$. Now suppose that E reveals a set S of signs, let l_1 denote the probability or likelihood that disease D_1, when known to be present, will give rise to sign S with similar likelihoods $l_2, l_3 \ldots l_n$ for the alternatives, then after examination E, Bayes's rule gives the final probabilities, $w_1, w_2, w_3 \ldots w_n$, called the posterior 'post-examination' probabilities that $D_1, D_2, D_3 \ldots D_n$ are correct as—

$$w_1 = \frac{p_1 \, l_1}{T} \qquad w_2 = \frac{p_2 \, l_2}{T} \qquad w_n = \frac{p_n \, l_n}{T}$$

where $T = p_1 + p_2 \, l_2 + \ldots p_n \, l_n$

As an example

Suppose a child A has been admitted with abdominal pain and the diagnosis suspected lies between one of non-specific abdominal pain, acute appendictis, mesenteric adenitis, or intussusception:
Then n, the number of possible diagnosis is 4, so

D_1 is 'non-specific abdominal pain'.
D_2 is 'acute appendicitis'.
D_3 is 'mesenteric adenitis'.
D_4 is 'intussusception'.

Taking figures at random, suppose that before examination it is 30 per cent probable that the child has non-specific abdominal pain, 10 per cent probable that he has acute appendicitis only, and only 1 per cent probable that he has mesenteric adenitis:
Then $p_1 = 0.30, p_2 = 0.10, p_3 = 0.01$, so that $p_4 = 1 - (p_1 + p_2 + p_3)$ $= 0.59$. That is the prior probability that an intussusception is present is 0.59.

Now let S denote the physical signs of a particular type observed during examination E. Suppose:
90 per cent of those children suffering from non-specific abdominal pain exhibit S ($l_1 = 0.9$)
50 per cent of those suffering from acute appendicitis exhibit S ($l_2 = 0.5$)
99 per cent suffering from mesenteric adenitis exhibit S ($l_3 = 0.99$)
10 per cent suffering from intussusception exhibit S ($l_4 = 0.10$)
Then T being equal to $p_1 \, l_1 + p_2 \, l_2 + \ldots p_n \, l_n =$
$0.3 \times 0.9 + 0.1 \times 0.5 + 0.01 \times 0.99 + 0.59 \times 0.10 = 0.3889$

$$w_1 = \frac{0.3 \times 0.9}{0.3889} = 0.69$$

$$w_2 = \frac{0.1 \times 0.5}{0.3889} = 0.1286$$

$$w_3 = \frac{0.01 \times 0.99}{0.3889} = 0.0225$$

$$w_4 = \frac{0.59 \times 0.10}{0.3889} = 0.1517$$

with $w_1 + w_2 + w_3 + w_4$ equal to unity which is correct. In other words, examination and the elicitation of the physical signs of disease has pushed up the probability of non-specific abdominal pain from 30 per cent to 69 per cent while that of acute appendicitis has increased only fractionally from 10 to 13 per cent. The probability of mesenteric adenitis has more than doubled but is still small at 2½ per cent and the chances that an intussusception is present has fallen from 59 to 15 per cent.

The doubt hanging over the Bayes theorem is the requirement of allotting the prior probabilities p_1, p_2 . . . p_n and until this is resolved Bayes's rule is unacceptable to the purist.

Nevertheless, the theorem has been made to work in the field of surgical diagnosis provided the database is built from a large enough number of representative cases and the clinical history, examination and subsequent investigations of the patient are accurately recorded. In the majority of systems that have been described, following entry of the information into the computer, a printback of the case history precedes the computer printout of the diagnostic probabilities.

Accuracy of computer diagnosis

1   *Applied to acute abdominal pain*

In the series analysed by de Dombal and his colleagues the overall accuracy of computer diagnosis was significantly higher in six out of eight disease categories. For example, of the 200 cases of acute appendicitis included in the sample the clinician, usually a registrar or senior registrar, diagnosed 88 per cent correctly whereas the computer diagnosed 99 per cent correctly. This disparity between the clinician and the computer in terms of accuracy of diagnosis was most dramatically shown in the diagnosis of diverticulitis when the clinician was accurate in only 50 per cent whereas the computer was correct in 100 per cent! The overall computer error in this total series of 304 patients was 8.2 per cent compared with 20.4 per cent for the clinicians.

It is also possible for the computer to assess the probability of a given disease so that the clinician is able to reconsider the necessary treatment. This may be of considerable importance; for example, in the distinction between acute cholecystitis and acute pancreatitis, because many surgeons are adopting a more aggressive attitude to the former, advocating cholecystectomy in the acute stage, whereas for acute pancreatitis, particularly in the early stages, treatment is becoming increasingly conservative. Thus, in the latter, laparotomy is now rarely performed and has been replaced in many centres by peritoneal lavage. Another function that can be performed by a properly programmed computer is to suggest further diagnostic procedures or an additional diagnosis, either of which could be valuable.

2   *Applied to jaundice*

Recently, the King's College group developed a computer programme capable of distinguishing between 11 different causes of jaundice. The

11 causes they considered in their programme included the three common 'surgical' causes; gall-stones, secondary hepatic metastases, and tumours of the extrahepatic biliary tree, together with 8 medical causes that included active chronic hepatitis, cirrhosis, acute viral hepatitis, drug-induced hepatitis, fulminating hepatic failure, primary biliary cirrhosis, and congenital hyperbilirubinaemia.

To assess the accuracy of such a computer diagnosis it was compared in each new patient to the final diagnosis, arrived at as a result of investigations such as liver biopsy, laparotomy, clinical follow up and, in some patients, postmortem examination.

The database for this investigation was provided by 309 patients suffering from jaundice, up to 72 items of information being obtained from each patient. Data from each new patient was selected on a sequential basis by the computer program according to its power to discriminate between the different diseases, using the particular results in that patient, until a final diagnosis was obtained. The data used from new, undiagnosed patients was only that which could be obtained within the first 48 hours after admission. This included 37 items derived from the clinical history, 12 from the physical examination and 23 from the subsequent haematological and biochemical investigations (72 items in all).

This group used the information and the computer in two ways: first, to establish the probability of one of the eleven diseases listed above, and secondly, to make a distinction between a 'medical' or 'surgical' cause of jaundice.

The results obtained by this group were as follows—

(a)   the computer diagnosis agreed with the final diagnosis in 66 per cent of the 219 patients;

(b)   the computer diagnosis of surgical versus medical jaundice was correct in 83 per cent.

Various explanations were advanced for the relatively poor results achieved in (a) above, one of the most valid of these being the inclusion in the database of large numbers of patients suffering from fulminating hepatic failure, in the treatment of which this group is particularly interested.

Since the Bayesian approach mimics, at least partly, aspects of the human mind's diagnostic process it became obvious that cases the clinician found easy to diagnose were diagnosed with equal certainty by the computer.

Other fields in which computer-assisted diagnosis has been assessed include, thyroid swellings, congenital heart disease and inflammatory bowel disease.

The following questions remain, however—

1   Do clinicians really need a computer aided diagnostic system?
2   Do such systems offer any measurable advantage over more conventional methods?

It is beyond any doubt that the construction of a database, because it is such a time-consuming feature of the system and demands such complete accuracy in the recording of data, greatly improves the clinican's performance, certainly during the time when he or she is working on its construction. Whether or not this enhanced performance outlasts the period of intense mental discipline required during the construction period is open to question.

It is possible that the increased use of computer-based diagnostic methods would help to reduce the ever-increasing number of investigations performed prior to surgery, for the problem of 'diagnostic overkill' is one of considerable importance at the present time when the financial resources of the health service are annually diminishing.

3 Urology

3.1 THE AETIOLOGY, DIAGNOSIS AND MANAGEMENT OF INJURIES AFFECTING THE KIDNEYS, URETERS AND BLADDER

Injuries involving the upper and lower urinary tract are relatively uncommon. It has been estimated that an average district general hospital will admit only four to five closed renal injuries a year. The number of closed injuries, particularly to the upper renal tract, following aircraft crashes is relatively high, and the incidence of penetrating injuries to the upper and lower urinary tracts is greatly increased in areas and cities in which stabbing is common.

CAUSATION OF INJURIES TO THE UPPER RENAL TRACT

(a) Closed injuries:
Road traffic accidents
Sports injuries
Aircraft crashes

(b) Open or penetrating injury:
Stab wounds
Gun shot wounds

(c) Iatrogenic injuries:
Retrograde catheterisation
Nephrolithotomy
Accidental avulsion
Renal biopsy

The frequency of closed injuries of the kidneys is higher in adolescent and young adult males because of the direct blows sustained to the loin in body contact sports such as rugby. Renal injuries, like splenic injuries, are commoner in the presence of pre-existing disease, especially a pre-existing intrarenal hydronephrosis.

Pathology of blunt injuries

(a)	Extrarenal	avulsion or damage to the renal pedicle
(b)	Intra-renal — minor:	contusion without capsular rupture.
	major:	laceration with associated capsular and calyceal involvement, the most severe injury of this type produces the so-called 'shattered' kidney.
(c)	Perirenal	associated with the development of a subcapsular and pericapsular haematoma.

Symptoms and signs

In about a third of all cases of blunt upper abdominal trauma the renal injury is associated with other injuries, particularly of the liver or chest which themselves may dominate the clinical picture.

The classical sign of a renal injury in the presence of an appropriate clinical history is the development of macroscopic haematuria. Severe bleeding, particularly from a shattered kidney, may result in hypotension and, in the renal angle, a palpable mass which may visibly increase in size within a few hours.

Haematuria may be absent if—

(a) the pelvi-ureteric junction has been avulsed;
(b) the ureter becomes obstructed by blood clot;
(c) traumatic occlusion of the renal artery occurs;
(d) when urine output is temporarily depressed by the development of haemorrhagic shock.

From the clinical standpoint renal injuries may be divided into mild and severe, and while the initial severity of the haematuria is not specifically helpful in distinguishing between these two broad groups, it is obvious that hypotension, in the absence of an associated abdominal or chest injury or the development of a palpable mass in the loin, indicates that a severe injury has occurred, such injuries being considerably rarer than the mild.

According to various series reported in the literature two-thirds of all closed injuries are mild, and of the remaining third only about 50 per cent require surgical intervention.

Management

Some aspects of the closed renal injury are still disputed, but those about which there is no disagreement include—

(a) The necessity of establishing as soon as possible the general condition of the patient and the presence of associated injuries. In particular, the blood pressure and pulse rate should be measured and regular observations made thereafter. If the renal injury is merely one facet of the clinical problem a central venous catheter line will probably be necessary (*see* Surgical Tutorials I, p. 13) and priority given to the most life-endangering aspect of the injury.

(b) The haemoglobin concentration should be determined and blood taken for grouping and cross matching.

(c) An intravenous infusion is required, at first using a 'neutral' solution such as Hartmann's, to be later followed by blood, if this is necessary.

(d) An intravenous pyelogram together with nephrotomography should be performed, perferably using a high dose of contrast medium.

Pyelographic findings

On the initial control film the following abnormalities may be visible—

1 Fractures of the lower ribs or transverse processes of the lumbar spine.
2 A lumbar scoliosis.
3 Loss of the psoas shadow.
4 Varying degrees of deformity of the renal outline due to perirenal extravasation.

On the excretory films the important findings are—

1 a normally functioning kidney on the side opposite to the lesion;
2 no change on the affected side—this indicates a mild injury;
3 the presence of filling defects in the collecting system or enlargement of the renal outline, indicating the presence of blood clot;
4 absence of some or all of the collecting system together with an extravasation of dye, indicating destruction of the affected part of the kidney;
5 total absence of function on the affected side which may be due to—
   (a) complete disruption of the kidney,
   (b) avulsion of the kidney,
   (c) thrombosis of the renal artery.

Retrograde catheterisation is now deemed of little value and carries the risk of introducing infection into a perirenal haematoma.

There is still some disagreement, particularly between the British and American surgical schools, as to the advisability or otherwise of renal angiography. The majority of British surgeons would consider renal angiography totally unnecessary in the majority of patients in whom, following admission, the blood pressure and pulse rate remains stable and the haematuria shows signs of diminishing within 48 hours of admission.

If, however, surgery is indicated, either because intravenous pyelography fails to demonstrate any function on the affected side or there is obvious deterioration accompanied by a rapidly developing mass in the renal angle then, assuming facilities are available, renal angiography would be deemed helpful. This investigation may help to indicate whether some form of conservative surgery is possible or whether nephrectomy is the only possible alternative.

In contra-distinction to the conservative views of the British School many American surgeons argue that renal angiography is a necessary investigation in all patients suffering from renal trauma. There can be little doubt that it will provide the most accurate anatomical information concerning the extent of the injury but whether such accuracy is really needed in the majority of cases remains debatable. Furthermore, except in the rare case of renal avulsion, it is doubtful whether angiography helps to predict which apparently clinically stable patients will require delayed exploration.

Surgical exploration

When exploration of an injured kidney is deemed necessary the transperitoneal approach is considered by the majority of surgeons to be superior to the extra-peritoneal approach because the renal pedicle can be more easily identified and controlled early in the course of the operation.

One of three surgical manoeuvres may be required, depending on the severity of the renal injury; repair of a cortical laceration, partial nephrectomy, or nephrectomy.

Late results

(*a*)   in mild or moderate injuries in which near normal pyelograms were initially obtained, a return to normal within a few weeks can be expected.

(*b*)   with severer renal damage, residual pyelographic changes are common; these include areas of calcification, calyceal diverticuli, non-functioning segments and, rarely, complete infarction which leads to total non-function on the affected side.

Surgical interference following apparent recovery is occasionally required to deal with a perinephric abscess, encapsulated collections of urine and, occasionally, the development of a pararenal pseudohydronephrosis.

URETERAL INJURIES

The great majority of ureteric injuries are iatrogenic, approximately one half following gynaecological operations and the remainder conservative or radical excision of the rectum. Rarely, the urologist may inadvertently damage the ureter during the removal of a stone by a Dormier basket or similar instrument.

Treatment

1   *Damage to a ureter recognised at the time of surgery*

This injury can be treated by the following methods—

(*a*)   by immediate re-anastomosis of the cut ends of the divided ureter after adequate spatulation (fishtailing) of the two ends of the ureter to provide an oblique anastomosis;

(*b*)   if the ureter has been divided low down so that reanastomosis is impossible, the upper end of the ureter should be re-implanted into the bladder.

Numerous techniques have been described to accomplish this, including the Boari flap (Fig. 3.1), the psoas hitch of Turner-Warwick. Alternatively, a uretero-ureterostomy can be performed anastomosing the damaged ureter to the ureter on the opposite side.

2   *Delayed recognition*

This is more likely than immediate recognition. When bilateral damage has occurred the patient fails to pass urine. If the damage is unilateral, the patient continues to pass urine but develops increasing pain in the loin and, finally, a urinary fistula develops, usually per vaginum following a gynaecological procedure, or following an abdomino-perineal resection through the perineal wound.

Once a fistula has formed the diagnosis can be established by the intravenous injection of methylene blue. Treatment is directed to re-implantation, although the results are generally reported to be less satisfactory than those that follow immediate recognition and repair.

BLADDER INJURY

This occurs in three ways—

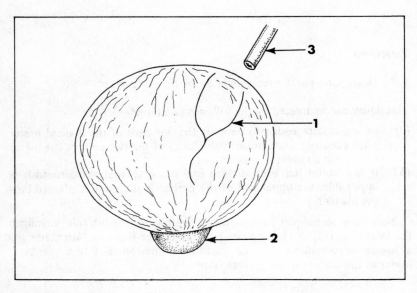

Fig 3.1 (A) Construction of Boari flap
1. Bladder incision   2. Prostate   3. Ureter

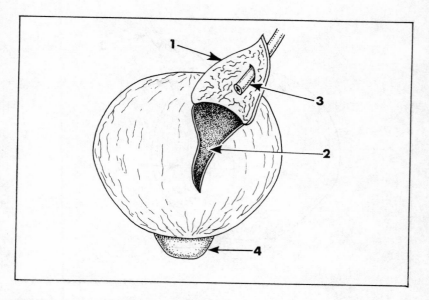

Fig 3.1 (B)   Construction of Boari flap
1. Flap turned over to reveal mucosa on inner surface   2. Interior of bladder
3. Ureter brought through flap below apex   4. Prostate

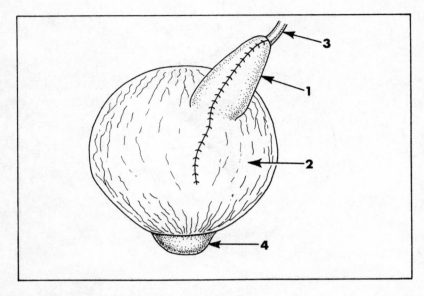

Fig 3.1 (C)   Construction of Boari flap
1. Boari flap completed   2. Bladder   3. Ureter entering flap   4. Prostate

1   **Intraperitoneal rupture**

Aetiology

(a)   This type of injury usually follows a blow to the lower abdomen at a time when the bladder is full.

(b)   Iatrogenic injury, which may occasionally follow—

   (i)   diathermy treatment of a bladder tumour;
   (ii)   resectoscopic treatment of tumours;
   (iii) the Lockwood repair of a femoral hernia.

Most intraperitoneal ruptures involve the fundus and posterior surfaces of the bladder because, as the bladder distends with urine, so the anterior surface becomes partially devoid of its peritoneal covering whereas the reflection from the pouch of Douglas remains in situ.

2   **Extraperitoneal rupture**

Aetiology

This type of rupture occurs in approximately 10 per cent of all cases of fractures of the pelvis and is commonly the result of a laceration of the bladder by a spicule of bone derived from a fractured pubic or ischial ramus. Although the empty bladder is not immune from such injuries it is more common when the bladder is partially or wholly distended. The majority of these injuries involve the anterolateral bladder wall, usually close to the bladder neck. Extensive extravasation of urine may occur, the extravasating fluid diffusing into the tissues of the anterior abdominal wall, the upper thighs, and even the buttocks, due to its escape from the pelvis via the greater sacrosciatic notch.

3   **Combined intra- and extraperitoneal rupture**

This type of injury is usually due to a missile or severe pelvic injury caused by crushing and is frequently associated with rectal injuries.

Diagnosis

Intraperitoneal rupture

The diagnosis of many intraperitoneal ruptures is made chiefly on the history and the suspicion that such an injury may have occurred. Because uninfected urine causes little peritoneal irritation evidence of peritonitis may not be present for at least 48 hours. After this, however, the development of an ileus, associated with fever and leucocytosis, indicates that there has been an intra-abdominal catastrophe. Following a large tear, no urine will be passed per urethram from the time of the accident onwards. Smaller tears may be successfully sealed by adherence of the omentum to the laceration, but when the diagnosis is suspected and the physical signs are insufficient to justify immediate laparotomy a cystourethrogram performed under strict aseptic conditions may verify the diagnosis.

Extraperitoneal rupture

When an extraperitoneal rupture has occurred the patient may, in the early stages, continue to pass blood-stained urine. If, however, a patient suffering from a fractured pelvis fails to pass urine and develops increasing tenderness in the suprapubic region an extraperitoneal bladder rupture should be suspected. The diagnosis can be confirmed by cystography using a water soluble medium which will cause little or no irritation of the tissues into which it will inevitably leak if the diagnosis is confirmed.

Treatment

Intraperitoneal rupture

The classical method of management of intraperitoneal rupture is immediate laparotomy and, after ensuring that there is no concommitant injury to other structures, suture of the tear in two layers, leaving an indwelling urethral catheter in situ for 14 days.

Extraperitoneal rupture

As with intraperitoneal rupture, the classical management of extraperitoneal rupture of the bladder is immediate exploration, cystostomy, and closure of the defect when once it has been isolated. Recently, however, papers have appeared suggesting that this type of injury can be equally successfully treated by the use of an indwelling urethral catheter left in situ for a period of 4 to 6 weeks, depending upon the presence or absence of associated injuries.

3.2 THE AETIOLOGY, DIAGNOSIS AND MANAGEMENT OF URETHRAL INJURIES

Urethral injuries may be open or closed and involve any part, i.e. the penile, bulbous, membranous or supradiaphragmatic portions.

Aetiology

Penetrating wounds at any point along the urethra are rare in peace time but become common in war when they are usually the effect of missiles or landmines. In civilian life, an occasional open injury will be the result of a stab wound. Closed injuries occur from a type of injury, 'straddle type', which causes damage to the bulbous urethra, or in association with fractures of the pelvis which result in tears at the junction of the membranous with the prostatic urethra.

Injuries to anterior urethra

The straddle type injury is the result of the individual falling astride an object or, alternatively, being kicked in the perineum. The pelvis may remain intact or, if sufficient force is applied, a unilateral or bilateral fracture of the pubic and/or ischial rami may occur.

In either event the urethra is injured by compression between the offending object and the inferior border of the symphysis.

Diagnosis

The diagnosis is usually obvious. Clinical examination reveals painful bruising of varying degree in the perineum and, if the mucous membrane of the urethra has been injured, blood will be seen at the external meatus. X-rays of the pelvis may or may not show evidence of bony injury.

This type of injury can be followed by extravasation of urine into the fascial compartment of the scrotum and perineum which, in turn, leads to necrosis of the subcutaneous tissues and overlying skin. Subsequent infection results in gangrene.

Management

1 Attempt to pass a narrow-bore catheter such as a Gibbon's. If this can be done with ease and clear urine is obtained from the bladder it should be left in situ for a period of 10 to 14 days, by which time the urethral wall will have healed.

Stricture formation can be expected, but in this position it can normally be treated by bouginage at ever-extending intervals of time.

2 If a catheter cannot be passed into the bladder in order to prevent increasing extravasation, a suprapubic cystotomy should be performed. If necessary, the perineal haematoma should be drained in order to diminish tissue tension and so prevent tissue necrosis.

Again, such treatment will normally be followed by a stricture which may be treated by intermittent dilatation. Should the stricture be so severe that its treatment by dilatation drastically curtails the life-style of the individual, urethroplasty should be advised.

3 In some centres, following suprapubic cystotomy, the patient is placed in lithotomy and the perineum is deliberately explored with the object to excising, if possible, the torn ends of the urethra, and performing a primary suture. This form of treatment is, however, rarely practised in the UK.

Injuries to the posterior urethra

Apart from iatrogenic injury caused by ill-judged or difficult instrumentation the commonest cause of posterior urethral damage is accidental trauma.

Crushing injuries of the pelvis may be associated with fractures of ischial and pubic rami with or without subluxation or complete disruption of the symphysis pubis and the sacroiliac joints. When such a severe injury has occurred the initial management is often dominated by the subsequent hypovolaemic shock caused by blood loss and the associated injuries.

The urethral injury itself involves the junction of the prostatic and membranous portions of the urethra and it is rare for the true prostatic, the true membranous, or the intradiaphragmatic parts of the urethra to be injured.

Diagnosis of posterior urethral injuries

The diagnosis of a posterior urethral injury should be suspected when—

(a) an injury is accompanied by a fracture of the pelvis, particularly when the pubic or ischial rami are broken or the symphysis is separated;

(b) the patient cannot pass urine following an injury associated with a fractured pelvis;

(c) a tender suprapubic mass is present;

(d) rectal examination reveals a freely mobile prostate the apex of which can be readily pushed up by the examining finger, Vermooten's sign. This sign can be misleading, however, if the prostate is difficult to palpate due to haematoma formation.

The diagnosis of a posterior urethral rupture can be confirmed by—

(a) the passage of a soft rubber or latex catheter. The withdrawal of clear urine excludes a complete but not an incomplete tear;

(b) retrograde urethrography;

(c) urethroscopy.

However, while each of these manoeuvres is possible, their advisability and the overall management of posterior urethral injuries has been the subject of argument for many years.

Management

The problems associated with posterior urethral injuries include—

(a) the resuscitation of the severely injured person;
(b) the management of associated injuries, e.g. of bladder and/or rectum;
(c) technical problems in effecting restoration of the urethral lumen and thus diminishing the length and severity of the ensuing stricture;
(d) imperfect understanding of the mechanisms relating to urinary continence;
(e) the management of the bony injuries.

There are two schools of thought regarding the treatment of posterior urethral injuries in patients in whom physical examination discloses that prostatic dislocation has not occurred. The first, the chief protagonist of which is J.P. Mitchell, is that the urethral injury should be left undisturbed and a suprapubic cystotomy performed. Mitchell believes that in the type of accident most commonly seen today, in which the injury is caused by impact, as in the road traffic accident, as opposed to crushing, the urethra is often split rather than completely divided, and that incomplete rupture is more common than complete. Mitchell argues that the remaining bridge of urethral tissue can only be harmed by the passage of a catheter and that not only may an indwelling catheter lead to necrosis of the remaining urethral bridge but also to infection of the pelvic haematoma.

Mitchell suggests that a urethrogram should be performed after 10 days in order to confirm the nature, site, and severity of the injury and then, at 21 days, the urethra should be visually inspected taking great care not to produce false passages by using a direct viewing instrument.

The opponents of this view consider, however, that a narrow soft blunt catheter should be introduced and, assuming that urine is obtained, it should then be left in situ for one to two weeks, after which it can be removed and a urethrogram performed to establish the severity of the injury. It should, however, be remembered that if a catheter is passed and no urine is obtained the explanation may be that—

(a) the bladder is empty, particularly likely if an associated intra-peritoneal vesical rupture has occurred;
(b) the catheter has passed into the retropubic space;
(c) hypotension may have led to temporary suppression of urine formation.

When physical examination reveals that the prostate is dislocated a number of different manoeuvres have been described. They include—
1 Aligning the urethra by the passage of a Foley catheter. This cannot be done unless the injured area is exposed by opening the retropubic space. Once this space is opened and the apex of the prostate is identified, a Foley catheter is introduced via the external meatus, and when identified as being in the pelvis it is led into the torn proximal urethra. If this proves

impossible, the older technique of 'railroading' the catheter into the bladder must be attempted. The problem then remains of obtaining as much approximation as possible between the two ends of the torn urethra. Initially, once the Foley catheter had been introduced, a period of traction on the catheter used to be advised in the pious hope that this would bring the torn ends of the urethra into apposition, albeit imperfectly. However, this technique is liable to produce damage to the bladder neck and urethra and has been abandoned.

2 An alternative technique more commonly used at the present time is to insert a series of stitches between the capsule of the prostate and the upper layer of the pelvic diaphragm. Alternatively, non-absorbable sutures can be passed from the perineum upwards, through the pelvic diaphragm and into the substance of the prostate, and then downwards once more to emerge in the perineum. Such stitches, when tied, approximate the prostate to the pelvic diaphragm and are left in place for a period of two weeks.

3 If the general condition of the patient is satisfactory and there is no associated rectal injury, some surgeons advocate the much more radical approach of repairing the injury immediately by exposing the injured area in a transpubic approach. Symphysiotomy has, of course, been used for many years by the obstetricians and was first introduced by Sigault in 1777. In 1972, Pierce described total pubectomy as a means of exposing the prostatic and membranous parts of the urethra in dealing with post-traumatic strictures, and in the Vietnam war this type of operation was in fact used for the repair of missile injuries involving the posterior urethra. The symphysis is divided by a Gigli saw, after which it can, in the young adult, be spread to a distance of 8 to 10 cm by means of a rib retractor. The bladder is then opened and a Foley catheter introduced per urethram. Once the haematoma has been removed further bleeding is controlled, after which the prostate and urethra are so mobilised that the torn ends can be brought into apposition. As an incidental finding it was shown that traction on the Foley catheter, when introduced into the bladder at the time of operation, did not bring about the apposition of the torn urethra as had been theoretically anticipated, and it was found that such apposition could be obtained only when the neck of the bladder and prostate has been mobilised from their ligamentous moorings.

Once the urethral defect is repaired the symphysis is allowed to fall together, the Cave of Retzius is drained, and the catheter retained in situ for 10 to 18 days.

Complications of posterior urethral injuries

The immediate complications of posterior urethral trauma are—

(a) pelvic sepsis, which is particularly likely when there is associated rectal damage, even if a proximal colostomy is performed at the time of operation and antibiotics are administered immediately;

(b) Osteitis pubis, producing disabling pain and a shuffling gait caused by loss of abduction due to spasm of the adductor muscles.

The late complications include—

(a) stricture formation which may required some form of reconstructive surgery, page 217;

(b) impotence.

3.3 AETIOLOGY AND MANAGEMENT OF URETHRAL STRICTURE

Since strictures of the urethra are virtually confined to the male, this tutorial will be limited to a discussion of their aetiology and management in the male.

ANATOMY OF THE MALE URETHRA

The urethra of the adult male is between 18 to 20 cm in length. It is divided into three parts, the prostatic, membranous, and spongy or penile portion. In the flaccid state it forms a double curve and, except during the passage of fluid, is normally a mere slit; in the prostatic portion it is crescentic, with the convexity ventral, in the membranous part stellate, and in the spongiose portion, transverse, the external meatus lying in the sagittal plane.

(a) *The prostatic urethra,* approximately 3 cm long, runs almost vertically through the prostate from the base to the apex. On the posterior wall is a median longitudinal ridge which is formed by the urethral crest. The floor of the prostatic urethra is perforated by the orifices of the prostatic ducts and at or about the middle of the urethral crest is the colliculus seminalis. On this is the slit-like orifice of the prostatic utricle on each side of which is the opening of an ejaculatory duct.

(b) *The membranous urethra* is the least distensible and shortest portion of the urethra and with the exception of the external meatus is also the narrowest. It descends, with a slight ventral concavity, surrounded by the muscle fibres of the external sphincter, through the perineal membrane to a point approximately 2.5 cm postero-inferior to the pubic symphysis. On either side lie the bulbo-urethral or Cowper's glands.

(c) The spongiose portion of the urethra begins in the bulb of the urethra which is closely applied to the inferior fascia of the urogenital diaphragm. It first continues the concave curve of the membranous urethra to a point anterior to the lowest level of the symphysis pubis, and from that point in the flaccid state curves downwards. This portion of the urethra has a uniform diameter of about 6 mm apart from the bulbous dilatation at its origin and the terminal position in the glans known as the navicular fossa.

The lumen of the spongiose portion of the urethra is lined by pseudo-stratified columnar epithelium from the fossa navicularis proximally to the membranous urethra, and except at its most anterior part presents the orifices of numerous small mucous glands and follicles, the urethral glands. There is no muscularis mucosa or other support for the surface epithelium and only a thin layer of loose connective tissue separates the mucosa from the spongy tissue and the smooth muscle.

In the membranous urethra the epithelial lining is transitional cell in type and a thick submucous layer of collagen and elastic fibres replaces the blood sinuses of the spongy urethra. Prominent layers of smooth muscle, inner longitudinal, and outer circular, spread up from the perineal membrane into the prostate, apparently bringing the lumen under muscular control.

AETIOLOGY OF STRICTURE

The aetiology of urethral strictures in the Western world has altered considerably in the past three decades because—

(*a*) gonorrhoea can now be controlled by the use of antibiotics, if the patient can be persuaded to attend for treatment;

(*b*) the increasing use of endoscopic prostatic resection has led to an increasing number of iatrogenic strictures.

In consequence, whereas thirty years ago most strictures were due to the long-term effects of Neiserian infections they are now mainly due to instrumental or accidental trauma.

CLASSIFICATION

I   CONGENITAL

II   ACQUIRED

A   Inflammatory: Postcircumcision meatal stenosis
Postgonoccal
Non-specific urethritis
Tuberculous
Urethral chancre

B   Neoplastic: Urethral carcinoma

C   Traumatic: (1) Accidental
(2) Iatrogenic: (i) Instrumental following cath-eterisation or endoscopic resection
(ii) Postoperative following retro-pubic prostatectomy or amputation of penis

212

Congenital strictures

These are rare. The commonest are found at the meatus but occasional strictures are met with at the proximal extremity of the fossa navicularis and in the membranous urethra.

A more frequent cause of urinary obstruction in the infant is narrowing of the preputial orifice following recurrent attacks of ammoniacal dermatitis, a condition commoner in bottle-fed than breast-fed babies because of the slight alteration in the pH of the stools of the former that favours the growth of an organism capable of splitting urea to ammonia. In such infants, if the prepuce is removed and the underlying condition is left untreated, an acquired meatal stricture may develop.

Acquired strictures

Postgonococcal. Whereas this type of stricture is becoming increasingly uncommon in the Western world it still remains the commonest cause of stricture in some African countries, notably Uganda.

Pathology

Postgonococcal strictures vary in length from mere diaphragms to strictures which involve the greater part of the bulbous and, occasionally, the penile urethra. The disposition of such strictures is related to the distribution of the paraurethral glands which are greatest in number in the proximal parts of the urethra where they extend into the corpus spongiosum, whereas in the penile urethra they are relatively infrequent except in the area proximal to the meatus.

During an acute attack of gonorrhoea, urethroscopy reveals pus issuing from the orifices of these glands and at the height of the infection the microabscesses that form in the glands rupture into the corpus spongiosum, thus permitting urinary extravasation to occur during micturition.

However, bacteria are seldom found in an established stricture unless there is a urethral fistula, or secondary infection of the urinary tract. It has been suggested that the importance of infection lies in the squamous metaplasia it subsequently induces, since microscopic examination of postgonococcal strictures always shows that the affected area is lined by squamous epithelium external to which is a thick collagenous layer. While the strictured area itself often shows little evidence of inflammatory change, inflammation is evident proximal to the stricture.

The hypothesis has been advanced that squamous metaplasia is important because after such a change the urethral lining becomes relatively inelastic. As a result, because the mucosa is unsupported it is liable to rupture during voiding, thus permitting urinary extravasation, which causes submucosal inflammation. This then heals with accompanying fibrosis, and as this increases in degree so the lumen eventually becomes encircled and a stricture is created.

213

Extensive gonococcal strictures are always made up of a series of rings of scar tissue, separate and distinct or confluent, which become progressively tighter and thicker towards the proximal end of the urethra. Proximal to the stricture the urethra is dilated, and the mucosa is often affected by areas of hyperkeratosis and increased pigmentation.

Complication of postgonococcal strictures

The chief complication associated with postgonococcal strictures is the development of multiple perineal fistulae. These follow extensive rupture of the mucosa proximal to the stricture or instrumental trauma. Either allows urine to leak into the spongy tissue, which is followed by secondary infection and the formation of periurethral abscesses which, after pointing in the perineum, lead to the typical 'watering can' scrotum.

Traumatic strictures

(*a*)   *Straddle injury*

This type of injury is caused by the bulbous urethra being crushed between the inferior border of the pubic arch and an object, e.g. a hurdle, over which the patient has fallen astride. Incomplete or complete tearing of the urethra may occur. This injury is associated with considerable perineal bruising and blood may appear at the external meatus.

(*b*)   *Complicating fractures of the pelvis*

Urethral injuries occur only when the pubic and ischial rami or the symphysis pubis, together with their associated ligaments, have been damaged. The incidence of urethral injury following road traffic accidents varies between 5 and 10 per cent according to the series examined, but all patients admitted suffering from pelvic fractures must be assumed to have sustained a urinary tract injury until proved otherwise. There exists, however, a rough correlation between the degree of such injury and the expectation of urethral damage, patients sustaining fractures of both pubic rami having a significantly higher incidence of urethral damage than those patients suffering from only a single fracture, and wide symphyseal separation is also particularly significant.

This type of injury is virtually limited to the male because the shortness and relative mobility of the female urethra renders it a more mobile structure.

The male urethra is usually injured at the junction of the prostatic urethra with the membranous and, if the tear is complete and the puboprostatic ligaments are completely disrupted, the prostate is displaced upwards and backwards by the development of the subsequent haematoma. Such injuries are always associated with ecchymosis and bruising of the perineum, together with extravasation of urine into the extraperitoneal perivesical space.

Regardless of the primary treatment a severe stricture nearly always follows this type of injury.

Iatrogenic strictures

1   *Post-catheterisation*

Strictures of variable length may be produced by the use of indwelling urethral catheters when these are—

1   left in the urethra for too long;
2   the calibre of catheter is of too large a diameter for the urethra;
3   complicated by urethral infection.

Such strictures may be limited to the external meatus, the proximal extremity of the fossa navicularis or, when there has been severe urethral infection, almost the entire length of the urethra may be involved.

2   *Following endoscopic manipulation*

The use of too large an endoscope may result in injury to the urethra, especially in the region of the penoscrotal junction, at which point, once the instrument has been passed into the bladder, the urethral mucosa is subjected to considerable pressure. Mucosal necrosis and subsequent extravasation lead inevitably to fibrosis. In one large reported series the incidence of stricture following transurethral prostatic resection was approximately 6 per cent.

Such strictures can be avoided by—

(*a*)   initial calibration of the urethra to determine the optimum size of the endoscopic sheath that should be used;
(*b*)   gentle dilatation before introducing the resectoscope;
(*c*)   adequate lubrication;

(d)   meatomy, or occasional perineal urethrostomy, in order to introduce the instrument with ease;

(e)   reducing the size of the catheter used for postoperative drainage to 24F or less.

3   Postprostatectomy strictures

Strictures following retropubic prostatectomy are relatively uncommon. Those that occur may be situated at the external meatus, along the length of the penile urethra, both the result of catheter damage, or at the junction of the prostatic urethra with the membranous. The most important factor appears to be the use of an indwelling catheter in the postoperative period but surgical trauma accounts for the majority of strictures met with at the junction of the prostatic with the membranous urethra.

Narrowing of the bladder neck may occur following retropubic prostatectomy but this is not considered to be a true stricture since resection of the offending bar usually resolves the problem permanently and completely.

4   Following amputation of the penis

Strictures are relatively common following either partial or complete amputation, the stricture developing at the mucocutaneous junction.

Clinical history of urethral stricture

The clinical history of an individual suffering from a urethral stricture is commonly dominated by the aetiological factor. However caused, all strictures eventually result in difficulty of micturition, hesitancy, and a diminished strength of the urinary stream. In the presence of infection, dysuria follows and, later, stone formation. In the latter stages, should the stricture go untreated back pressure effects on the kidneys results in renal failure.

Investigation

The specific investigations required prior to starting any form of treatment include—

(a)   Biochemical: Blood urea.

(b)   Haematological: Haemoglobin and erythrocyte count.

(c)   Radiological.

1   *Urethrography*

The whole of the urethra can be visualised by a combination of retrograde and voiding urethrograms. Such techniques also permit an assessment of sphincter involvement, if present, and also the visualisation of false passages and fistulae.

2   *Intravenous pyelography*

Since a stricture acts like any other obstructive lesion of the lower urinary tract the specific complications associated with back pressure can ultimately be expected. Pyelography may reveal—

(*a*)   Distension of the bladder and postmicturition retention.
(*b*)   Hypertrophy and sacculation of the bladder wall.
(*c*)   Diverticuli of the bladder.
(*d*)   Changes in the upper urinary tract, including bilateral hydronephrosis.

3   *Urethroscopy*

This should be performed using a direct viewing instrument, although such an examination is of limited diagnostic value because it allows an inspection only of the stricture *en face*. It may, however, play a distinct role in therapy by enabling a filiform bougie to be passed into the stricture and then onwards into the bladder.

Techniques of treatment

The method of treating a particular stricture depends upon many factors including—
(*a*)   the age and general condition of the patient;
(*b*)   the aetiological factor;
(*c*)   the site;
(*d*)   the response to conservative therapy.

1   *Conservative therapy: Urethral dilatation*

Intermittent dilatation is usually performed by passing plastic bougies, with or without the use of a leading filiform, which may be passed:
(*a*)   by manipulation,
(*b*)   by the 'faggot' method,
(*c*)   under direct vision, using a urethroscope.

Unfortunately, the passage of a filiform bougie through the distal face of a stricture does not necessarily mean that it will pass along the whole length of the stricture, particularly if this has been complicated by the production of false passages caused by previous failures. The aim of dilatation should be to dilate the stricture with the minimum of trauma and discomfort.

Occasionally, dilatation of a difficult stricture requires the use of sounds. If the strictured area is in the bulb, help in passing a metal sound can be obtained by placing the patient in the lithotomy position and inserting the index finger of the left hand into the anus in order to guide the sound through the strictures and into the bladder, an assistant holding the shaft of the penis over the sound.

The two major hazards following dilatation are—

(*a*)   the creation of false passages,

(*b*)   the occurrence of bacteraemic shock.

Meatal strictures, e.g. following the use of too large a catheter after prostatectomy, may be expected to resolve after treatment by intermittent dilatation, whereas the majority of strictures elsewhere in the urethra normally continue to need intermittent dilatation throughout the life of the patients.

2   *Internal urethrotomy*

This procedure, in common use in the past for the treatment of post-gonococcal strictures, is now having a resurgence of popularity due to the development of a direct vision instrument, although, following urethrotomy, intermittent dilatation is still required.

3   *Urethroplasty*

The use of plastic procedures is determined by—

(*a*)   the age of the patient;

(*b*)   the frequency with which dilatation is required;

(*c*)   the frequency of bacteraemia and bacteraemic shock following dilatation;

(*d*)   the presence of complications such as fistulae.

The results of reconstructive surgery can be expected to be better when the stricture has been caused by injury rather than infection because in the former the remaining urethra is normal both in calibre and structure whereas the precise extent of postinflammatory strictures may be very difficult to determine.

The surgeons who have made major contributions to reconstructive urethral surgery include Denis Browne, Turner-Warwick, Swinney

Johanson, and Blandy. Particularly with regard to the repair and reconstruction of strictures in and above the membranous urethra, the chief point of disagreement lies between the protagonists of one- and two-stage reconstructive procedures.

The one stage island patch technique (Figs 3.2, 3.3) has been particularly advocated by Blandy. In this operation the floor of strictured area is excised along its whole length up to the level of the veru montanum, and immediately replaced by a patch of scrotal skin which is obtained from the tip of a scrotal flap that has been raised to expose the urethra. This ellipse of skin relies for its blood supply on its attachment to the dartos muscle, an attachment that is carefully maintained once the patch has been separated from the main flap.

The advantages claimed for this operation are that it avoids the long delay of several months which occurs between the first and second stages of a two-stage repair. However, many surgeons would argue that although there is an inevitable delay in a two-stage procedure, during the whole of which the patient must micturate sitting down through what is in reality a perineal urethrostomy, it has one significant advantage, i.e. after the first stage is completed and the scrotal flap has been sutured to the floor of the divided urethra, examination at intervals of two to three months enables the surgeon to determine that the whole of the strictured area has been excised and that the second stage will, therefore, be successful (Fig. 3.4).

In practice, most urethroplasties are performed for posterior strictures of traumatic or inflammatory origin and, so far as the former are concerned, the first stage seldom requires revision prior to a closure of the perineal defect by remobilisation of the scrotal flap. The final result of the two-stage procedure depends upon the stability of the calibre of urethra prior to final closure, and if this is in doubt the operations must be revised.

When it is necessary to carry the scrotal flap as high as the veru montanum it might be thought that the interference with the external sphincter might cause incontinence. However, Turner-Warwick who has made a special study of this aspect of the problem states that it is a relatively rare complication. He and others have shown that continence at resting bladder pressures requires only an intact bladder neck sphincter or an intact musculo-elastic mechanism in or immediately above the membranous urethra, one or other being sufficient.

More recently, Blandy has described a transpubic approach to strictures involving the bulbous and membranous parts of the urethra. This method appears promising and, furthermore, logical.

Complications of posterior urethroplasty

1 The commonest complication is restenosis. It is a particularly common hazard following the treatment of post-inflammatory strictures.
2 The development of a hairball due to the continued growth of hair in the inlaid skin.

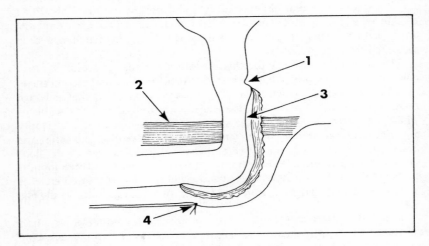

Fig 3.2   One stage urethroplasty – saggital section
1. Verumontanum   2. Pelvic diaphragm   3. Pedicled island graft cut from full thickness
of scrotal skin flap and maintaining blood supply from connection with dartos muscle
4. Resutured scrotal skin: posterior portion deprived of dartos to provide blood supply
to graft

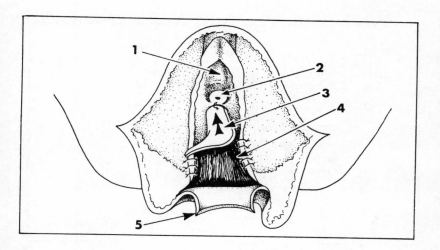

Fig 3.3   One-stage urethroplasty – as seen from perineum as partially completed operation. The island graft is about to be sutured at its anterior end to the posterior extremity of the anterior urethra
1. Roof of urethra   2. Verumontanum   3. Direction in which flap is sutured   4. Pedicle of dartos   5. Scrotal skin stripped of dartos

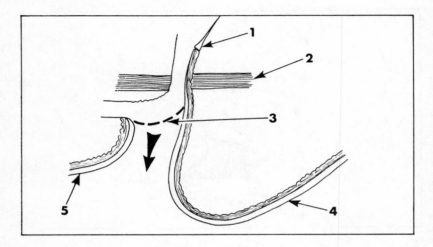

Fig 3.4 (A)   Two-stage urethroplasty in saggital section – Stage I
1. Verumontanum   2. Pelvic diaphragm   3. Floor of stricture removed   4. Scrotal flap
with underlying dartos muscle brought up to the level of the verumontanum   5. Scrotal
skin and dartos muscle sutured to anterior urethra

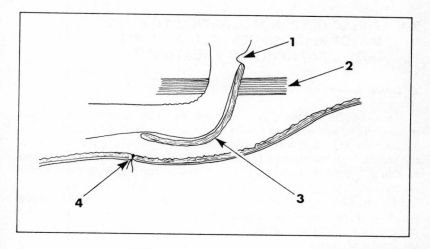

Fig 3.4 (B)   Two-stage urethroplasty in saggital section – Stage II completion of repair
1. Verumontanum   2. Pelvic diaphragm   3. Skin flap separated from excess of scrotal skin and sutured to the posterior extremity of divided anterior urethra   4. Continuity of scrotal skin restored

3 Leakage following micturition is particularly likely if the diameter of the reconstructed urethra exceeds that of the normal so that a pool of urine can collect within it.

4 Pseudo-wetness. If the skin flap retains its normal sensitivity the patient may feel a sense of wetness in the perineum, even though there is no leakage, due to urine flowing over the inlay.

5 Fistula formation.

3.4 THE UNDESCENDED, RETRACTILE AND MALDESCENDED TESTIS; DIAGNOSIS, COMPLICATIONS AND TREATMENT

Testicular descent

The role of the various factors concerned in the descent of the testes remains uncertain. For many years it was believed that the gubernaculum, a fibromuscular cord, actively contracted, thereby pulling the testes into the scrotum. However, since this structure at its distal end is only attached to skin it is unlikely to be able to exert any meaningful degree of traction on the testes. It is now generally agreed that the gubernaculum is formed from a mere broad band of undifferentiated mesenchyme which creates a pathway of least resistance along which the testes pass, possibly pushed by positive intra-abdominal pressure and, possibly, by the milking action of the cremaster muscle.

There are three phases of testicular descent—

1 *The relative phase.* This is the result of the differential growth rate of the metanephros, which ascends dorsal to the developing gonad, pushing this organ caudally as it does so. This phase in the human is believed to be completed within 55 days.

2 *Transabdominal movement.* This is believed to arise due to enlargement of the liver and kidneys which causes an increase in the intra-abdominal pressure thereby pushing out the processus vaginalis. This, in turn, exerts traction on the developing gubernaculum and pulls the testes to the internal ring, a process completed within 150 days.

3 *The inguinal passage.* The gubernaculum immediately distal to the testes and within the inguinal canal swells. This dilates the canal, thus permitting the increasing intra-abdominal pressure to push the testes onwards from behind. Once within the canal it is believed that the gonads are fairly rapidly propelled downwards by the action of the external oblique muscle so that descent is completed at some time between the seventh month of intra-uterine life and birth.

Experimental and embryological studies suggest that testicular descent is controlled by the testes' own production of testosterone under the influence of chorionic and, possibly, fetal pituitary gonadotrophin.

Non-descent

Three categories of non-descent (cryptorchism) were described by Hinman.

1 Those associated with *abnormalities of the gubernaculum or inguinal canal.* This leads to failure of descent of an otherwise normal testis.

2 *The dysgenetic testis.* This testis is grossly and histologically abnormal. Approximately 20 per cent of all undescended testes belong to this group, and the importance of recognising it lies in the fact that, in such males, 30 to 60 per cent of the contralateral testes will also be abnormal.

3 *Deficient hormonal stimulation.* Lack of hormonal stimulation commonly leads to bilateral non-descent.

Retractile testes

In addition to failure of descent a testis may also be retractile, i.e. it may be pulled into the upper scrotum or even into the lower inguinal canal by a hyperactive cremaster muscle. A retractile testis is often mistaken for an undescended testis, particularly if the affected child is examined in a cold environment.

Maldescent

The testis having traversed the inguinal canal in a normal fashion comes to lie in an abnormal site, commonly in the superficial inguinal pouch, less commonly in the suprapubic region, and rarely in the perineum.

Incidence of cryptorchism

The true incidence of undescended testes was established by Scorer in 1964 when he examined 3600 infants and found the incidence of non-descend at one year was unlikely to descend thereafter. The explanation to 0.8 per cent at the end of one year.

Since the adult incidence of crytorchism is accepted as being between 0.2 and 0.8 per cent, Scorer concluded that a testis which had failed to descend at one year was unlikely to descend thereafter. The explanation of other previous reports suggesting that a large number of testes descended after the first year is that these series included significant numbers of retractile testes.

The probable reason spontaneous descent occurs in the first year of life is because of the effects of gonadotrophins carried over from fetal life. These hormones are in high concentration from the seventh month of intrauterine life until birth and then decline to very low levels until the tenth year. They then increase to a peak again at puberty and after this decline slowly towards middle age. This supports the theory that a hormonal stimulus is necessary for normal descent, and a further piece of evidence in favour of this theory is the high incidence of nondescent in premature infants, which has been found to be as high as 27 per cent.

Position of the undescended testis

The majority, 70 per cent, of undescended testes are situated in the inguinal canal and only about 25 per cent are abdominal or retroperitoneal. The remaining 5 per cent are ectopic or completely absent.

Associated conditions

1   *Inguinal herniae*

In most babies suffering from undescended testes a patent processus vaginalis is present even though the sac is often too narrow to permit the descent of the abdominal contents. If the hernia is clinically evident at first examination of the child it forms an indication for immediate operation to prevent the potential danger of strangulation.

2   *Trauma*

Whereas ectopic testes are definitely at risk, an inguinal testis is only a little more in danger than its scrotal counterpart.

3   *Torsion*

Undescended testes are more likely to undergo torsion than the normal because of their abnormal vascular and serous attachments. Torsion of an abdominally retained testis is rare; in adults this complication is of graver significance than in the child because it is preceded by malignant change in approximately 60 per cent of patients.

4   *Malignant change*

The incidence of nondescent in cases of testicular tumour, as found by retrospective study, is between 5.9 to 14.3 per cent. The risk of tumour development in an undescended testis is put at 30 to 50 times that of a testis in the normal position. The bilateral cryptorchid is particularly at risk since if a tumour develops on one side, the chance of malignancy in the opposite testis is 1 in 4.

The 'prune belly syndrome'. In this condition the lower abdominal muscles are absent, leading to a typical deformity in the lower abdomen. The syndrome is commonly associated with bilateral crytorchism, together with abnormalities of the urinary tract, especially dilatation of the bladder.

6   *Psychological effects*

The importance of this is open to doubt. Various authors have quoted differing opinions, some considering that the child becomes increasingly disturbed between the ages of 3 and 6 years of age by the absence of a testis or testes. Such an argument can be used in favour of surgical treatment between these ages.

An important point from the surgeon's viewpoint is that orchidopexy does not appear to lessen the risk of malignant change in the testis that is brought into the normal position. Furthermore, almost 20 per cent of testes which become malignant are the contralateral normally placed testes. This fact suggests that the abnormal position is not in itself the carcinogenic agent, but rather that there is a primary testicular defect responsible for both nondescent and the increased risk of malignancy. The only value of orchidopexy is that a tumour developing in a scrotal testis is more easily diagnosed and, therefore, theoretically at least can be treated at an early date.

However, the incidence of testicular tumour in the male population is only 2.1 per million so that the problem posed by undescended testes is relatively insignificant.

Functional changes in the undescended testis

Histological changes occur in the tubules of undescended testes and infertility follows. Testosterone production may be affected but the individual usually achieves full sexual maturity with all secondary sexual characteristics present, together with adequate potency. Only exceptionally will the bilateral cryptorchid be fertile.

Electron microscopic studies suggest that changes begin in an undescended testis at the age of 3 years and routine microscopy shows positive abnormalities at 6 years of age.

The cause of the tubular changes that are accompanied by inadequate spermatogenesis remains to be finally determined. These are two hypotheses—
(*a*)   changes in the environmental temperature of the undescended testis.
(*b*)   that the structural changes are of congenital origin.

Whereas there is a considerable difference of opinion with regard to the initial changes that take place in an undescended testis, all investigators agree that there is a decrease in tubular size, a decreased number of spermatogonia and, lastly, that gross interstitial fibrosis develops by the time of adolescence. These changes result in the affected testis becoming much smaller than its normal counterpart, the change being particularly marked after the age of six.

TREATMENT OF THE UNDESCENDED TESTIS

It is now generally agreed that if an undescended testis is obviously associated with a congenital hernia, orchidopexy and herniotomy should be performed immediately. In the absence of any obvious hernia, the age at which operative intervention should take place has gradually diminished. This is particularly so during the past two decades because of the increasing appreciation of the tubular changes that take place in the abnormally sited testis.

Hormonal treatment

This form of therapy was introduced in 1931, using human chorionic gonadotrophin (HCG), a hormone that is produced in the placenta and found in both the blood and urine of pregnant women. In the female, its action is predominantly that of the pituitary luteinising hormone, and in the male it stimulates the interstitial cells of the testes and consequently the secretion of androgens. Various courses have been suggested, 500 to 1500 units once or twice daily for 4 to 8 weeks, 500 units twice weekly for 6 weeks and, latterly, a short course of 3300 units on alternate days for 6 days. At first, extravagant claims were made for the efficacy of hormonal treatment and even as late as 1938 it was being reported as successful in 65 per cent of bilateral and 47 per cent of unilateral cases of cryptorchism. Only later was it appreciated that many of these apparently satisfactory results had been obtained in patients suffering from retractile testes.

It is now the general opinion that hormonal treatment is only worthy of trial in cases of bilateral cryptorchism. The optimum age for starting treatment appears to be between 2 and 5 years and a success rate of only about a third can be expected. It has been pointed out by some observers that the fertility in those patients with bilateral cryptorchism who respond to HCG is greater than those who require surgery, but this is not unexpected since a proportion of those children not responding to hormone therapy will possess dysgenetic testes the function of which is unlikely to be improved by surgery.

Surgical treatment

At present, orchidopexy is usually performed before the child enters school at the age of five years. The essential operative features of orchidopexy are—

1 Dissection of the spermatic cord from its surroundings so that the cord as a whole may be lengthened sufficiently to allow the testis to lie without tension within the scrotum. A hernial sac, if present, is divided above the testis, dissected from the cord and ligated at the level of the deep inguinal ring. Difficulty encountered in removing the sac from the cord can be minimised by infiltrating the cord with saline, thus separating its various parts.

2 Cord lengthening. If, after careful dissection of the cord, the testis cannot be brought into the scrotum, several techniques may be attempted:

(*a*) Division of the suspensory ligament of Browne. This is composed of a group of fibres, which radiate upwards and laterally from the cord at the level of the deep inguinal ring, and are best seen when the cord is drawn downwards and medially.

(*b*) Further lengthening can also be achieved by incising the medial edge of the internal ring and so taking the 'kink' out of the cord. There is no indication to divide the inferior epigastric artery which can usually be displaced medially.

(*c*) A further technique that may lengthen the cord is division of the spermatic artery itself which leaves the viability of the testis dependent upon the vasal vessels. This method is theoretically possible if the former can be divided at a sufficiently high level to preserve an anastomosis between the two systems.
   Prior to such action the spermatic artery should be temporarily occluded in order to be certain that the testis remains viable. Since the length of the artery rather than the vas forms the limiting factor in 'cord length', microvascular techniques have recently been described in which the origin of the spermatic vessels is brought lower down the aorta.

3 Fixation of the testis. The older operations, such as that described by Torek, in which the testis is temporarily fixed, by implantation into a subcutaneous tunnel to the thigh have now been generally abandoned because the tension created normally led to a high incidence of testicular atrophy. It is now more common to fix the testis within a subcutaneous pouch formed by dividing the fascial layer, which is identified by a finger from within the scrotum.

If the testis, despite the manoeuvres described previously, cannot be satisfactorily brought into the scrotum it has been suggested that it should be fixed at the lowest point attainable without undue tension and then re-explored some time in the future when cord lengthening according to the advocates of this procedure will have occurred. However, the author has never found this satisfactory; usually at the second operation the testis is merely surrounded by scar tissue.

Results of orchidopexy

(a) *Testicular atrophy*

The incidence of testicular atrophy following orchidopexy has been variously reported at between 2 to 50 per cent. However, many of the results from which these figures were obtained were from older series in which undue strain had been placed on the testicle by placing it in the thigh.

(b) *Fertility studies*

Fertility studies, although difficult to perform, show a variation in results between 30 to 70 per cent.

(c) *Percentage paternity ratios*

This is defined as the percentage of married patients who have become fathers. In a recent study in which 112 patients who had undergone orchidopexy were traced (a response rate of 54 per cent) it was found that the paternity rate for patients in whom a unilateral orchidopexy had been performed was equal to that of a normal individual, whereas when bilateral orchidopexy had been performed the percentage was considerably less.

Orchidectomy

Assuming that the opposite testis is normally placed in the scrotum, orchidectomy becomes an acceptable method of treatment of the undescended or maldescended testis if it cannot be brought into the scrotum. However, in cases of bilateral non-descent it is as well to bury the testis deep to the external oblique until the position on the opposite side has been properly established. This, at least, ensures that testosterone formation will occur, which will result in the development of the normal secondary sexual characteristics.

3.5 PHYSIOLOGY, AETIOLOGY AND TREATMENT OF THE NEUROGENIC BLADDER

NEUROLOGICAL ASPECTS OF BLADDER FUNCTION

Central control

Central control of bladder function is exerted by cortical, subcortical, and spinal centres.

(a) Cortical centres

These are situated in Areas 4 and 6 and the main effect of the cortex is inhibitory. Since the bladder has bilateral cortical representation a unilateral lesion has little or only transient effect. Bilateral cortical lesions affecting the frontal or parasagittal areas produce an uninhibited bladder, the function of which resembles that of the infant before development of controlled micturition.

(b) Subcortical centres

Centres probably situated in the pons and medulla have both facilitatory or inhibitory influences. Release from the inhibitory effect produces a micturition reflex which is stimulated by a very reduced bladder volume.

(c) Spinal centres

Some doubt still exists as to the precise tracts down which the descending fibres travel, but there is complete agreement that there are synaptic connections in the lumbosacral segments. These are collectively known as the 'spinal micturition reflex centre'. When these centres are destroyed, particularly those of the sacral group, the bladder is deprived of reflex function and it must then rely on the intramural vesical nerve plexus which normally communicates with the spinal cord by way of both afferent and efferent fibres.

Afferent pathways from the bladder travel in the sympathetic, parasympathetic and pudendal nerves. Afferent stimuli are eventually interpreted as sensations of distension and pain.

Efferent pathways reach the bladder via the following routes—

(a) *Sympathetic outflow* is derived from the 2nd, 3rd and 4th lumbar segments, the fibres of which synapse in the inferior mesenteric ganglion. The postganglionic fibres then travel in the hypogastric nerves to the bladder. These nerves have little or no effect on bladder function but their destruction abolishes ejaculation in the male.

(b) *Parasympathetic outflow* reaches the bladder via the nervi erigentes from the 2nd, 3rd and 4th sacral segments. Stimulation of these nerves produces a strong contraction of the detrusor muscle and, conversely, section produces a flaccid paralysis.

(c) *Somatic efferents* derived from the 1st and 2nd sacral segments supply the pelvic floor and the striated muscle of the urethra. Whereas stimulation of these nerves produces elevation and closure of the bladder neck, section of the pudendal nerves does not lead to incontinence.

SPINAL SHOCK

Any injury that produces an acute transection of the cord, regardless of the level or whether the lesion remains complete or, in due course, is incomplete, is followed immediately by spinal shock. This may last from eight days to eight weeks during which all reflex activity is depressed and an imbalance between the facilitatory and inhibitory aspects of bladder control is present. The bladder does not respond to distension and, therefore, there is no desire to micturate, both the detrusor and skeletal muscles being flaccid. If the bladder is allowed to become grossly distended, overflow develops because the strength of the detrusor is not sufficient to overcome the partial blockage of the bladder exit. The duration and the effect of spinal shock depend upon—

(a)   bladder function prior to injury;
(b)   the number of disrupted spinal segments;
(c)   the age of the patient;
(d)   efficient management entails at this stage avoiding over-distension and infection.

The particular bladder syndrome that develops after the stage of spinal shock depends upon—

(a)   level of spinal cord lesion;
(b)   completeness or incompleteness of lesion;
(c)   whether there was mechanical urinary obstruction before the injury.

INFLUENCE OF NEUROLOGICAL LEVEL OF LESION

(a)   Transection proximal (above) the spinal vesical reflex centres occurs when the cord is damaged above the second lumbar segment, which is equivalent to a bony lesion above the 10/11th thoracic vertebra. Because such a bladder is cut off from the facilitatory and inhibitory impulses it is known as the *automatic reflex* or *upper motor neurone bladder.*

When 'balanced', this type of bladder will spontaneously void its contents, because when it is sufficiently distended the sensory receptors in its wall evoke, through the afferents, a reflex contraction of the detrusor muscle with reciprocal relaxation of the various sphincter mechanisms.

Alternatively, voiding may be precipitated by a variety of stimuli, e.g. pressure on the suprapubic area, pulling the pubic hairs, hitting the thighs, or stimulation of the external anal sphincter.

In the early stages, the power of the detrusor contraction may be inadequate, particularly if there is any element of mechanical obstruction, and as a result residual urine develops. This is usually considered unacceptable if it becomes greater than 5 to 10 per cent of the full bladder capacity. In the absence of mechanical obstruction, inadequate detrusor function is particularly likely if the bladder is subjected to initial and prolonged over-distension in the stage of spinal shock or if infection develops.

Lack of balance between the afferent and efferent components of the vesical reflex arc may lead to either hypo- or hyper-reflexia, conditions made worse by irritable lesions elsewhere in the body or by organic changes in the bladder such as infection or hypertrophy of the bladder neck. A most troublesome bladder is one in which very little distension produces detrusor contractions; the result is a reflex incontinence. This type of bladder is known as the *uninhibited hypertonic cord bladder.* Once the bladder is hyperactive the afferent impulses may spread to involve all the isolated cord so that micturition is associated with either flexor or extensor spasms of the legs and even arms.

(*b*) Transection below the spinal vesical centres involving the conus medullaris or spinal nerves takes place when the spine is injured below the level of the twelfth thoracic vertebra. Such a bladder is completely isolated and should eventually become autonomous, depending for its contractile activity upon autonomic intramural innervation. This bladder is often known as the *lower motor neurone bladder.* Such a bladder cannot itself produce a powerful enough emptying contraction and it has therefore to be assisted or activated by contracting the abdominal muscles, which produces an increase in the intra-abdominal pressure. A patient suffering from such a lesion usually states that the bladder is emptied by extrinsic pressure and that voiding ceases when such pressure is reduced.

BLADDER MANAGEMENT

The initial management of the bladder has the following aims—

1 the prevention of infection;
2 the prevention of over-distension;
3 prohibiting over-enthusiastic manual expression which can lead to hydronephrosis or even deep vein thrombosis;
4 making the patient catheter-free as soon as possible.

The debate continues over the use of continuous or intermittent catheterisation in the early stages. The majority of spinal injury centres now appear to have abandoned continuous urethral drainage because of the high incidence of bladder infections and urethral strictures that follow. Even the small calibre Gibbon catheter with an overall diameter of 1.5 to 2 mm seems to be unsatisfactory.

In the Second World War, Riches introduced a new method of continuous suprapubic catheterisation, employing a small 16 F catheter, but this also leads to bladder infection, and even the smaller infantile peritoneal dialysis cannula, recently introduced by Cook and Smith, is not without similar hazards, although it has been adopted in some spinal centres.

Guttmann insists that intermittent catheterisation by a meticulous no-touch technique is the correct treatment and in his unit he was able to show that the urine of 70 per cent of males remained sterile, thus supporting his argument.

Guttmann's reasons for preferring intermittent catheterisation after 12 to 24 hours of the injury as opposed to immediate continuous drainage are—

1 Early drainage by an in-dwelling catheter even of the Gibbon variety may be followed by bladder infection within two to four days if not within 24 hours. Thus, he argues, there is really no difference in this respect between an in-dwelling urethral catheter and drainage by suprapubic cystotomy.

2 An important reason, he suggests, for using intermittent catheterisation is to allow the urethral mucosa to become gradually accustomed to a foreign body. The tone of all tissues, he argues, is greatly diminished in the state of spinal shock and, as a result, the threshold to pressure is lowered and injury to the mucosa facilitated.

3 In incomplete and complete cord lesions in young people, where an early return of reflex function can be expected, intermittent catheterisation encourages the physiological stimulus for micturition, i.e. some bladder distension sets up appropriate impulses to the spinal reflex bladder centre thus promoting an early return of detrusor activity.

The whole period during which catheterisation is necessary should be monitored by frequent inspection of the urine. Fresh specimens are examined and cultured, and if there is infection it is treated with an appropriate antibiotic of which there is now a wide choice.

LATE BLADDER MANAGEMENT

Once the stage of spinal shock is over, the bladder may remain 'unbalanced' and unable to empty properly. This is an indication for transurethral resection of the bladder neck, an operation first used in 1945 at the Mayo Clinic. The time to perform the resection remains a matter of debate. Some would advocate surgery as early as 2 to 6 weeks after the return of reflex spinal activity. Others would delay operation for approximately three months.

Resection is wholly successful in about 1 in 5 patients and the usual advice is to resect too little rather than too much. Resection of too much may render the patient incontinent, which is particularly serious in the female. Other operations designed to open up the bladder neck are the V-Y plasty, but such operations are difficult to repeat, if they are at first unsuccessful, because of scarring.

Features that draw attention to defects in bladder function are dribbling due to true or overflow incontinence, suprapubic pain, hesitancy, and the symptoms of infection such as fever, chills, dysuria, haematuria, and pyuria.

3.6 DIAGNOSIS AND MANAGEMENT OF RENAL TUBERCULOSIS

Deaths from renal tuberculosis have fallen in a dramatic fashion over the last three decades due to: (a) the control of bovine tuberculosis, (b) the use of antitubercular drugs, and (c) the effects of immunisation of tuberculin-negative children between the ages of 10 to 13 years with the living attenuated organism, the Bacilli Calmette Guerin.

Such has been the effect of these various factors that only some 20 deaths a year from renal tuberculosis have been notified in the United Kingdom in the last five years, and when death does ensue it is usually due to uraemia caused by renal destruction.

Clinical presentation

The disease may present in any one of five ways—
1 By symptoms related to the upper urinary tract, including increasing frequency of micturition due to tuberculous nephritis, aching in one or other loin, and haematuria.
2 By symptoms related to the lower urinary tract, including intense frequency, dysuria, incontinence, and severe haematuria.
3 By symptoms related to renal destruction, including the constitutional disturbances of uraemia, fatigue, loss of weight, and anaemia.
4 By genital lesions, i.e. chronic epididymo-orchitis.
5 By constitutional symptoms alone, including loss of weight, loss of appetite, and night sweats.

Pathology

Genitourinary tuberculosis is always secondary to a tuberculous focus elsewhere. Patients presenting with a genital lesion have a pre-existing lesion in the kidney in about 50 per cent of cases.

The basic pathological lesion of tuberculosis is the follicle or tubercle which forms after the initial acute inflammatory response to the organism is over.

Once the polymorphonuclear cells have been destroyed by the organisms there is a progressive infiltration of macrophages into the affected area. Most of the macrophages phagocytose the bacilli and change in character to epithelioid cells. Others fuse to form giant cells which have a granular eosinophilic cytoplasm with nuclei arranged in a peripheral ring or crescent. Surrounding this multitude of altered macrophages is a wider zone of small round cells which are mainly lymphocytes. Usually, within 10 to 14 days, there is a coagulative necrosis (caseation) in the centre of this cellular mass to complete the formation of the follicle. The caseous material is caused by allergy to tuberculoprotein, and it has the consistency of cream cheese. Once present it tends to attract lime salts, with the result that areas of calcification may develop in a tuberculous lesion.

In renal tuberculosis the kidneys are infected by haematogenous spread from a primary focus which may or may not be recognisable. Both kidneys are seeded with bacteria to produce a tuberculous 'nephritis', at which stage organisms may be found in the urine. Under favourable circumstances healing takes place, but in unfavourable conditions tubercles develop. These are usually confined at first to only one kidney, and the initial lesion is localised in the cortex or the corticomedullary junction. From this initial starting point the disease spreads towards the medulla. As the tubercles coalesce, cavities form in the renal tissue and the disease eventually breaks through to communicate with the calyces.

Continued spread leads to increasing destruction of the remaining calyces and papillae to produce the ulcero-cavernous stage. By this time, infected debris is continually being discharged into the urinary tract and the disease spreads downwards to involve the ureter and, eventually, the bladder, all the involved epithelial surfaces being eventually replaced by caseous tuberculous granulation tissue.

The narrower parts of the renal tract, i.e. the necks of the calyces, the pelvi-ureteric junction, or the ureterovesical junction may become obstructed by inflammation and associated oedema or, later in the disease if healing occurs, by fibrosis. Similarly, once the bladder is severely affected, apart from spasm, fibrosis may develop, leading to a bladder of such small capacity that the patient becomes incontinent. At this stage in the disease there is also vesico-ureteric reflux which accelerates the renal damage.

Genital tuberculosis in both male and female also commonly develops by haematogenous spread, but in the male there may also be direct spread. In the male, the prostate, seminal vesicles, and the epididymis become involved; in the female, a tuberculous endometritis or salpingitis may develop. At first a tuberculous epididymitis forms a tense, tender swelling which later becomes hard, painless and nodular. Later still, the skin becomes attached to the underlying structures and a sinus, which may discharge caseous material, develops.

Diagnosis

The investigations required in a suspected case of renal tuberculosis are—
1 Urine examination.
2 Radiological examination.
3 Cystourethroscopy.

Urine analysis

In all but advanced cases the isolation of the tubercle bacillus from the urine may be difficult and, occasionally unsuccessful, due to the intermittent excretion of organisms and the difficulty encountered in culturing the organism.

The classic finding is of a sterile pyuria, but this is not inevitable. Normally, three pooled early morning specimens are examined. The urine is collected in jars containing 2 per cent sodium hydroxide which destroys contaminating organisms. At the first examination only about 50 per cent yield a positive culture on Lowenstein's medium, indicating the intermittency of excretion. Guinea-pig inoculation can be performed but the necessity for this has been reduced by the recognition that multiple urine sampling should be used as a routine measure. The organism is stained by the Ziehl-Neelsen method, using hot carbol fuchsin.

Radiological examinations

1 *Plain X-rays of the abdomen and pelvis* may reveal granular, annular or homogeneous areas of calcification. The latter is observed particularly in the relatively rare tuberculous pyonephrosis. Prostatic calcification must be distinguished from calculi.

2 *Intravenous pyelography* may show—
(a) Lack of definition of a minor calcyx, indicating ulceration of the papilla.
(b) Dilatation of any part of the pelvi-calcyceal system, indicating obstruction.
(c) Cavitation. This is seen only when there is communication with the drainage system. Widespread cavitation indicates gross ulcerocavernous disease.
(d) Reduced or absent renal function.
(e) The ureters may appear irregular in outline due to the presence of mucosal granulations, stricture formation, or dilatation due to uretero-vesical reflux. Tuberculous structures are commonest at the lower end of the ureter.
(f) The bladder may be small and irregular in outline.

Cystography

(a) Micturating cystography may demonstrate free ureteric reflux due to incompetence of the diseased uretero-vesical junction.
(b) The bladder itself may form a thick soft tissue shadow around the dye, indicating thickening of the vesical wall. Either spasm or fibrosis may reduce the bladder capacity.

Chest

Active pulmonary tubercle may be present. In Europe, before the introduction of chemotherapy, one in twenty patients had an active lung lesion.

Cystoscopy

This investigation must be performed with extreme care if tuberculosis is suspected because sudden over-distension of the bladder may lead to bleeding from the diseased mucosa which obscures the view.

The mucosal changes are variable. The bladder may, of course, be normal, in which case the bladder capacity and the appearance of the mucosa are normal. Once the bladder is involved the capacity diminishes and the mucosa appears pink in colour. Occasionally, tubercles or ulceration may be seen. Severe contraction, the bladder holding only a few ml of fluid, is usually associated with the classic 'golf hole' ureteric orifice.

TREATMENT

Chemotherapy

In the preantibiotic era as many as 50 per cent of patients suffering from renal tuberculosis died within 5 years of the diagnosis, due either to advanced renal failure or severe extrarenal lesions.

With the introduction of triple therapy, streptomycin, isoniazid, and p-amino salicyclic acid, and the development of the second line antituberculous drugs, the mortality of this condition has fallen to less than 2 per cent.

In common with all antituberculous therapy the initial treatment for the first 3 to 6 months is carried out with all three drugs, after which isoniazid and PAS are continued for a further period of 18 months. At the present time, rifampicin is gaining in popularity as a substitute for streptomycin and PAS. It can be combined with isoniazid and ethambutol in alternating courses of two weeks duration for one year.

Surgery

During the preantibiotic era the standard treatment of renal tuberculosis was nephroureterectomy followed, after recovery, by a long period of convalescence. The sole indication for such radical surgery is now restricted to the patient presenting with total destruction of the kidney due to a tuberculous pyonephrosis. Otherwise, surgery is rarely indicated although some surgeons have advocated limited operations such as the drainage of local intrarenal abscesses.

Although renal involvement may lead to renal destruction, a commoner cause is ureteric obstruction. This usually follows healing of a tuberculous lesion in the ureter. The treatment of this complication is as follows.

Treatment of ureteric stricture

Steroids, e.g. prednisolone 20 to 30 mg daily in divided doses, have been used to try to prevent the formation of organic strictures during treatment in patients known to have ureteric involvement. However, these drugs are probably only effective when the ureter is still oedematous and it is unlikely that they are beneficial once a fibrous stricture has developed.

The majority of strictures develop at the lower end of the ureter. The site can be ascertained by a retrograde ureterogram using a Braasch catheter, which permits a regime of intermittent dilatation by a Braasch bulb dilator. This must be repeated at fortnightly intervals and the results followed by repeated intravenous pyelography.

Some regard this manoeuvre as completely ineffective and resort to immediate surgery if the obstruction is progressing or renal function is declining. If the bladder capacity is normal, the strictured lower end of the ureter can be excised and replaced by a Baori flap. If, however, the bladder is contracted, such a flap may be difficult or impossible to fashion, in which case the stricture is excised and a direct vesical implantation performed.

If this is impossible or the stricture is at a higher level the ureter must be excised and replaced by a length of ileum.

Any of these surgical procedures may be preceded by a nephrostomy but this should be avoided if possible because of the dangers of secondary infection.

Treatment of the contracted bladder

Gradual reduction of the bladder capacity by fibrosis may lead to incontinence and increasing renal destruction due to back pressure. Both of these undesirable side effects may be overcome by enlarging the bladder by an ileo-cystoplasty. If necessary, colon may be substituted for ileum, but which portion of bowel is used depends on the opinion of the individual surgeon.

Tuberculous epidydimo-orchitis

In the preantibiotic era, disease of epididymis nearly always eventually demanded orchidectomy or epidydimectomy. Direct surgery is now seldom used because once the diagnosis has been made triple therapy will usually control the disease and prevent sinus formation.

3.7 MEDICAL MANAGEMENT OF CALCULOUS DISEASE OF THE URINARY TRACT

The high recurrence rate following surgery for urinary stone has stimulated great efforts to solve the associated biochemical abnormalities. As a result it has been shown that in certain conditions specific treatment may reduce the recurrence rate. These conditions include—

1 Cystinuria

This is a rare condition and, therefore, stones composed of cystine are also rare. Such stones form in patients secreting a urine oversaturated with this compound, usually over 500 mg/day. Cystine crystals, hexagonal, white and translucent, can be seen in the urine, and the calculi are usually multiple, or form a cast of the calyces or pelvis. The urine is always acid. Two essential steps in treatment are to promote a diuresis by increasing the fluid intake, and to alkalinise the urine, which makes cystine more soluble. The latter is achieved by administering sodium citrate 20 g and potassium citrate 5 g, both dissolved in 100 ml of water and given orally in divided doses through the day.

More specific is the administration of D-penicillamine, which is a degradation product of penicillin. This is normally given in a divided daily dose of between 0.9 and 1.5 g. It acts by forming a soluble disulphide with cystine, thus preventing crystallisation in the urine. The toxic effects of D-penicillamine are headache, sore throat, fever and, occasionally, agranulocytosis. There is also a tendency to pyridoxine deficiency which can be prevented by the concomitant administration of vitamin B_6, 50 mg three times daily.

2 Uricosuria

Stones composed of uric acid are also rare. The pure uric acid stone is radiotranslucent, but the majority contain sufficient calcium oxalate to be radio opaque. They are usually multiple and facetted. Such stones are not necessarily associated with gout, and the level of uric acid excretion may be within normal limits, 0.2 to 0.5 g/24 hours.

Medical management of uric acid stone formation consists of—
(a) Restriction of protein intake to not more than 40 g a day because uric acid is an end product of purine metabolism.
(b) Alkalinisation of the urine by administration of sodium and potassium citrate.
(c) The use of allopurinol, dose 200 to 600 mg daily to inhibit xanthine oxidase which catalyses the conversion of hypoxanthine to xanthine and xanthine to uric acid. Although first introduced for the treatment of gout, it has been shown to be highly effective in the prevention of uric acid stone formation.

3 Hyperoxaluria

Primary oxaluria is caused by a defect in oxalate metabolism. In patients with hyperoxaluria, the endogenous production of oxalate increases, and large amounts of oxalate, 100 to 400 mg daily, are excreted in the urine as compared to the normal output of 15 to 20 mg, with the result that oxalate calculi are formed. No reliable method of dealing with this biochemical abnormality has yet been found but one of doubtful value is the use of pyridoxine, vitamin B_6. The biochemical rationale for this form of therapy is based on the knowledge that the vitamin acts as a coenzyme in the transamination reaction between glycine and glyoxylic acid.

4 Hypercalciuria

The normal daily calcium output varies between 100 and 300 mg. This is increased in certain well-defined pathological conditions which are associated with bone destruction, including, bone metastases, sarcoidosis, and hyperparathyroidism. In the last-named condition, the accepted treatment is removal of the offending tumour or hyperplastic glands, but if parathyroidectomy is contra-indicated, administration of ethinyloestradiol diminishes bone resorption, decreases the hypercalciuria, and thus delays growth or recurrence of the stone.

However, hyperparathyroidism is a relatively rare cause of stone formation. In the majority of patients who present with calcium phosphate/oxalate stones, which account for 90 per cent of all stones in the United Kingdom, the precise biochemical abnormality is unknown. However, investigation shows that excessive quantities of calcium are excreted in the urine, a condition known as idiopathic hypercalciuria. In order to reduce calcium excretion in this condition to within normal limits several suggestions have been put forward including—

(a) Dietary control of the calcium intake. A diet containing less than 200 mg of calcium leads to an output of between 130 and 180 mg Ca/24 hours.

(b) The effects of dietary restriction can be further enhanced by the concomitant use of a chelating agent such as ethylene diamine tetracetic acid, 0.5 g daily, or a binding agent such as sodium phytate, 125 mg/kg which forms an unabsorbable calcium complex in the gastrointestinal canal.

(c) An alternative method of reducing hypercalciuria is by the administration of thiazide diuretics. One that has been most extensively used is hydrochlorthiazide, 50 mg three times daily. Administration of this drug may reduce the total amount of calcium excreted by 50 per cent.

5 Phosphaturia

Phosphate is the second commonest radicle found in renal calculi. Its excretion can be altered by medication, but the end result appears to be indirect rather than direct. Thus, Edwards and his co-workers found that administration of disodium hydrogen phosphate dihydrate, 12 g daily in divided doses, increases the urinary excretion of phosphate, pyrophosphate, and citrate, but at the same time diminishes the excretion of calcium and magnesium. They demonstrated the favourable clinical effect of this type of therapy by showing that the number of stone-forming episodes in a group of recurrent stone formers was considerably reduced.

6 Infection

Renal tract infection may be caused by an anatomical disorder of the urinary tract or may follow the development of a stone. In either case, the precipitation of triple phosphate, calcium ammonium magnesium phosphate, is brought about either as a primary event or on a nucleus formed by a pre-existing stone. When an anatomical disorder is the cause of infection and stone formation, and is amenable to surgery, surgical correction of the abnormality should be attempted. When a stone forms in the absence of a specific anatomical abnormality the stone is removed, and following this one of the following measures may be helpful—

(a) *Acidification of the urine* by the use of ammonium chloride, 2 g three times a day. This reverses the alkalinity of the infected urine which predisposes to the precipitation of triple phosphate.

(b) *Administration of methylene blue,* 50 mg every four hours. This drug lowers the pH of infected urine and blocks the binding of ions by matrix. Even in the absence of infection, Boyce reported that this reduced the number and frequency of calcium oxalate/phosphate stones by almost 50 per cent.

(c) *Control of infection.* The most important aspect in preventing infective stones is to isolate the infecting organism and to suppress it by the appropriate antibiotic. For this to be successful, antibiotic sensitivity must be continuously monitored. Commonly used agents include, co-trimoxazole Tabs. 2, three times daily, carbenicillin BP, 250 mg four times daily, cephradine BP, 500 mg four times daily, and gentamicin 0.6 mg/kg body weight daily in divided doses.

4 Arterial and Venous Surgery

4.1 THE LATE RESULTS OF VARIOUS METHODS OF LOWER LIMB ARTERIAL RECONSTRUCTION

Arterial reconstruction, if possible, is indicated when the blood supply to the lower limb is—

(a) insufficient to allow the patient adequate mobility, i.e. severe intermittent claudication has developed;

(b) rest pain is present;

(c) examination reveals signs of incipient gangrene;

(d) minor degrees of gangrene are already present.

Statistically, only about 25 per cent of individuals presenting with the various symptoms of arterial occlusion actually require surgery; 15 per cent of the whole will eventually undergo amputation; and about 10 per cent die within a year of complaining of the symptoms of peripheral arterial disease from involvement of arteries elsewhere, either of the heart or the brain.

The common sites of occlusion are—

(a) the aorto-iliac region,—plaque formation with subsequent ulceration and thrombosis commonly occurs at the aortic bifurcation, and in the middle or at the bifurcation of the common iliac artery;

(b) the femoro-popliteal segment in which 70 per cent of the lesions occur at the adductor hiatus or in the adductor canal;

(c) the popliteal artery above the knee joint;

(d) the popliteal bifurcation.

Bilateral disease is commonplace, 70 per cent of patients with a femoro-popliteal occlusion having stenosis or occlusion in other limb vessels. Co-incidental proximal and distal occlusions are also common.

Investigation and various operations that have been designed to relieve this condition have been described in *Tutorial in Surgery I*, pp. 324–326, but here we are concerned only with the eventual prognosis following the various surgical manoeuvres already described. However, certain recent advances should be noted concerning—

1 *Diagnosis and localisation of the offending lesion*

(a) The use of Doppler ultrasound techniques is rapidly increasing and is especially useful in patients in whom clinical examination suggests that reconstructive surgery may well prove impossible. Thus, arteriography which is an invasive, and therefore potentially dangerous technique, can be reserved for those patients in whom there is a possibility of successful reconstruction. The parameters measured by ultrasound can be assembled to give a classification into three groups of the severity of the disease: a patent artery, a partly obstructed artery, and lastly, a totally obstructed artery with degrees of collateral circulation.

The parameters measured include the pulsatility index, the transit time, which requires two probes and the ability to record the signals from both simultaneously, and lastly, the damping factor, which is the ratio of the proximal to the distal pulsatility indices.

(b) ^{133}Xenon clearance, a method in which 0.1 ml ^{133}Xenon dissolved in isotonic saline is injected by means of a thin needle into the thickest part of the medial head of the gastrocnemius.

2 *Newer synthetic substitutes for femoro-popliteal bypass*

One of the newer materials is PTFE, expanded polytetrafluoroethylene. This compound offers certain theoretical advantages over other fibre prostheses. The graft consists of PTFE nodes interconnected by thin fibres which allow the ingrowth of tissue between the interstices and into the wall of the prosthesis so that a smooth intima is eventually formed on the inner surface. This is some 5 to 35 microns in thickness as compared with a thickness of 500 microns which is that of the intima forming on the inner surface of a Dacron graft. No preclotting of this type of graft is required since, unlike Dacron, no extravasation occurs even in a fully heparised patient because of the high PTFE to blood surface tension.

Results of Surgery

The results of arterial surgery can be assessed in a variety of ways. These include—

(a)   the relief of symptoms, of chief importance to the patient;
(b)   the incidence of complications;
(c)   patency of the system used;
(d)   subsequent necessity for amputation.

Endarterectomy

Advantages

In considering the various operations available endarterectomy would appear to have significant advantages over graft procedures in that it—

(a)   avoids transplantation of tissue or materials;
(b)   preserves all major branches of the segment of the artery that has been disobliterated.

Limitations

The method has, however, certain limitations including—

(a)   the need for an adequate run off from the disobliterated segment in order to prevent early thrombosis;
(b)   technical difficulties which usually occur when the atherosclerotic lesion is calcified or extends deeper than usual into the media; media;
(c)   the difficulty of its application to arteries in which the disease itself has caused contraction of the total diameter. This is now generally overcome by the use of autogenous vein patches.

Technique

Without doubt the major cause of late failure following endarterectomy is the involvement of the run off vessels distal to the extremely diseased segment which leads to a gradual diminution in the blood flow. When using endarterectomy several arteriotomies may be required and the distal intima must be tacked down prior to closing them. Furthermore, each arteriotomy may require closure by a vein patch because straightforward suture may reduce the calibre of the vessel which, in turn, has a great effect on the blood flow which is proportional to the radius, as stated in Pouiseuile's equation—

245

$$\text{Flow} = \pi\,r^4\;\frac{(p_1 - p_2)}{8\,\eta l}$$

in which r = radius, l = length, η = vicosity of the blood and $(p_1 - p_2)$ = pressure difference between the ends of the vessel.

The best results are achieved by endarterectomy when the artery is large, the occluded segment is short, and the diseased intima splits easily from the media.

Major difficulties are caused by extensive calcification or severe inflammatory change of the diseased vessel and under these circumstances it is generally agreed a graft yields better results. If it is considered that suture of the artery will produce reduction in vessel diameter then an autogenous vein patch should be used. In large vessels such as the aorta this problem seldom arises, the endarterectomy can be performed through a single longitudinal excision or, if the disease extends into the common iliac arteries, this incision can be directly extended on one side, although it is customary to leave a part of the wall intact on the opposite side if the disease is bilateral.

In vessels such as the common or superficial femoral, endarterectomy is performed through a number of arteriotomies using such devices as the Canon loop. In 1965, gas endarterectomy was described, in which carbon dioxide was injected under pressure into the arterial wall, the degree of stripping being limited by clamping the affected artery together with its branches. Whatever method is used the separated core is removed through the arteriotomy wounds.

Results

Aorto-iliac endarterectomy is a very satisfactory operation. Patency rates of over 80 per cent at 5 years have been repeatedly reported. Furthermore, in the majority of patients rest pain and intermittent claudication are abolished. These satisfactory clinical results are in parallel with the highly significant increase in the ankle systolic pressure (ASP) index after surgery, when normal values are often restored.

However, endarterectomy for disease of the femoro-popliteal segment is not so effective, the patency rate falling progressively as the patients are followed, hence at 0–6 months the accumulative patency is only as high as 60 per cent, and at 5 years approximately 30 per cent.

Profundoplasty

Recently, the operations of profundoplasty and extended profundoplasty have been performed. The former was first described by Martin and his colleagues in 1968, although the fundamental importance of the profunda artery in distal arterial disease had been recognised earlier.

In 1972, Martin and his colleagues suggested that profundoplasty might be used as an alternative to femoro-popliteal reconstruction because, being an artery of supply rather than of conduction, it is usually relatively free of atherosclerotic changes and, even when these do occur, they tend to be proximal rather than distributed along the whole length of the artery. This theme was developed by Cotton and Roberts who reported the use of an extended type of profundoplasty in 72 patients, in 69 per cent of whom femoro-popliteal reconstruction would have been possible. They reported that by performing this operation they were able to abolish intermittent claudication completely in approximately 50 per cent of patients and produce an extension of the walking distance to an acceptable 200 m in the great majority of them. Extended profundoplasty, however, means that the profunda artery, having been dissected free from its attachment is incised along its length until its wall is found to be supple. Following endarterectomy the subsequent defect is closed by an extensive vein graft. In a series of patients in whom bypass surgery would have been impossible they achieved a success rate of only 33 per cent and if distal gangrene was present only 25 per cent. Similar results have been reported by other authors even when the operation has been limited to a curved arteriotomy from the common femoral to the first major branch of the profunda, together with a local endarterectomy if the mouth of the profunda is found to be blocked at its origin.

The largest series of limited profundoplasty is that described by Martin and Bouhoutsos in 1977, in which they were able to review 112 patients in whom, in some, the operation had been performed at least nine years previously. In this series operative failure was deemed to have taken place if amputation was required prior to the patient leaving hospital, whereas a limited success was claimed if amputation was required within four years. In their entire series, satisfactory results were achieved in 68 patients out of a total of 107, in whom no amputation was required within 9 years.

Autogenous vein grafts

This operation was introduced by Kunlin in 1951 although the concept had been previously explored in the experimental animal by Carrel and Guthrie as early as 1905.

Technique

Normally, autogenous vein grafting is carried out by using the saphenous vein from the leg upon which the bypass is to be carried out. The saphenous vein, which should not be varicose, is carefully dissected out, tying all tributaries, from the level of the saphenous opening to the lower end of the thigh, and the proximal end is marked so that the operator cannot or will not forget to reverse the graft when the proximal anastomosis is made.

Results

The results obtained using autogenous vein grafts for the treatment of obliterative disease involving the femoral and popliteal arteries are appreciably better than those that follow endarterectomy in this area. Accumulative patency rates using this technique for the treatment of femoro-popliteal disease show that patency rates in excess of 60 per cent can be achieved. At 5 years the accumulative patency rate of vein grafts is of the order of 70 per cent whereas endarterectomy produces a patency rate of 40 per cent.

Factors affecting the result of a venous bypass

(*a*) Of considerable importance is the diameter of the vein. Grafts greater than 4 mm in diameter have a much greater patency rate some years after surgery than grafts of a lesser diameter.
(*b*) The run-off resistance. When this is high, the incidence of both early and late failures is increased but if all the vessels at the popliteal trifurcation are patent the success rate rises to 90 per cent.

Late bad results following vein grafting are nearly always associated with the worsening of the disease proximal to the graft.

Synthetic grafts

The use of synthetic grafts has been virtually abandoned except for disease of the aorto-iliac region and in this position a graft is nearly always used for the replacement of aneurysmal dilatation and not for obstructive disease. In aorto-iliac disease grafts of Dacron retain their patency over a long period, the 5-year patency rate varying in different series between 70 and 95 per cent. One problem associated with such grafts is continued aneurysmal dilatation proximally, or the occasional development of an aorto-duodenal fistula, the latter being a rare cause of haematemesis. The search, as indicated earlier in this tutorial for synthetic substitutes, continues unabated, particularly as certain miscellaneous operations that have been described for salvaging the lower limbs, in which autogeneous vein grafts were used have proved inappropriate because of the distances that must be covered.

These operations include—

(*a*) Axillo-femoral bypass grafts in which a graft is brought from the axillary artery to the femoral artery.
(*b*) Ilio-iliac anastomoses in which a graft is brought across the pelvis linking an unaffected artery on one side to a diseased artery on the opposite side.

Summary of factors affecting prognosis after arterial surgery

1 The pathological severity of the atherosclerotic condition, the degree of involvement of the arterial tree requiring reconstructive surgery, and the presence of disease elsewhere, particularly in the cerebral and cardiac circulations.

2 The site of the occlusion, the larger the vessel involved the better the result.

3 The length of the occlusion, the shorter the better.

4 The clinical stage the disease has reached before reconstructive surgery is attempted. Thus, the prognosis as regards the ultimate survival of the limb worsens at each clinical stage, i.e. claudication distance, rest pain, and gangrene.

5 Presence of factors predisposing to arterial disease, which include diabetes and hyperlipidaemia.

6 Type of surgical operation undertaken.

4.2 INDICATIONS AND RESULTS OF CORONARY ARTERY SURGERY

Coronary atherosclerosis is now so common that it represents the single most important cause of death in middle age in the industralised societies of the West. In the United States alone it is responsible for the death of 750,000 persons annually.

ANATOMY OF THE CORONARY CIRCULATION

The myocardium is supplied by two major arteries—

1   *Right coronary artery*

This arises from the anterior aortic sinus and emerges between the root of the pulmonary trunk and the right auricle to run downwards and to the right in the right portion of the coronary sulcus to the junction of the right and inferior surfaces of the heart, whereafter it turns to the left and runs on the posterior surface of the myocardium.

This is larger than the right coronary artery and arises from the left aortic sinus. It passes to the left and almost immediately divides into two major branches, a large anterior interventricular branch passing downwards towards the cardiac apex overlying the interventricular septum, and a left circumflex branch which passes round the atrioventricular groove to become the posterior descending artery.

The two arteries supply the two sides of the heart, and normally there is little, if any, anastomosis between them compared with the rich arterial anastomoses found in skeletal muscle.

Coronary flow

In a normal adult at rest the coronary flow is approximately 70 ml/min/ 100 g of myocardium, the normal weight of the myocardium being 300 g. Maximal exercise normally increases this flow between five- and six-fold to between 300 and 400 ml/min/100 g of myocardium, the vasodilatation permitting this greatly increased flow being largely mediated by the action of local metabolites.

CLINICAL SYNDROME OF ANGINA PECTORIS

The symptoms of angina were first described by Heberden in 1772 although it was not until 1912 that Herrich emphasised the association between atherosclerosis of the coronary arteries, angina, myocardial infarction, and sudden death.

The symptoms, easily recognised in about 70 per cent of patients, consist of intermittent attacks of retrosternal pain, each lasting seconds or minutes, which may be described as a feeling of 'pressure', 'constriction' or 'choking'.

Anginal pain commonly radiates upwards into the neck, and down the left arm in particular. In nearly every case the attack occurs during exercise or is preceded by emotional stress. Frequently, the patient spontaneously volunteers the information that the attacks are more frequent in winter or on sudden exposure to cold.

In some 30 per cent of patients the underlying pathology may go unrecognised because the symptoms are more suggestive of upper gastrointestinal disease such as a hiatus hernia, diffuse oesophageal spasm, or biliary colic. In some patients anxiety alone may precipitate similar symptoms in the total absence of organic disease.

Important factors in diagnosis

1 *Clinical features*

(*a*) The 'stress' factor. This should be evident from the clinical history and may operate either at work, in the home, or both.

(*b*) The duration and frequency of attacks. In the majority of patients the attacks last from a few seconds to a few minutes. If the pain persists for longer than 15 minutes myocardial infarction should be considered, since in the majority of patients once the precipitating factor of exercise or stress has been removed the pain spontaneously disappears. Relief may be hastened by the sublingual administration of glyceryl trinitrite. In a minority of patients the frequency and severity of the attacks increases to such a degree that the life of the afflicted individual is completely disrupted. This rapid deterioration, known as 'crescendo angina' frequently heralds the onset of infarction and it is particularly in this group of patients that coronary artery surgery should be considered.

2 *Clinical examination*

This may reveal little. Alternatively, it may reveal the presence of—

(*a*) hypertension and congestive heart failure;
(*b*) cardiac arrhythmia;
(*c*) signs of diabetes mellitus, e.g. glycosuria;
(*d*) signs of generalised atherosclerosis, e.g. absent pulses in one or both legs;
(*e*) tendon xanthoma or an unexpected arcus senilis;
(*f*) auscultation may reveal an apical fourth sound because of alteration in left ventricular compliance;
(*g*) Fundoscopy may reveal a retinopathy of diabetic or hypertensive type. In the former the retina is sparsely or thickly spattered with minute red dots which are microaneurysms. Larger blot and dot haemorrhages then appear followed later by waxy-looking exudates with harder edges than the cotton-wool patches seen in hypertension.

Hypertension may be associated with a variety of retinal changes all of which are dependent upon the duration and degree of the elevated blood pressure. In mild hypertension only narrowing of the retinal blood vessels may be seen whereas in severe hypertension papilloedema, together with increased haemorrhages and exudates occur. When these findings occur together in a relatively young patient they suggest the presence of Fredrickson Type II hyper β-lipoproteinaemia, familial hypercholesteraemia. This is an inherited, dominant, autosomal trait in which early coronary artery disease develops. The plasma is clear because the triglyceride fraction is normal or only slightly raised, the serum cholesterol is grossly elevated, and on electrophoresis the β-lipoprotein band which carries the cholesterol appears.

Specific investigations

1 Electrocardiography

(a) Approximately 50 per cent of patients suffering from angina have a normal resting ECG although minor nonspecific changes in the ST segment are relatively common.

(b) If an ECG is performed during an attack, transient ischaemic ST segment depression confirms the diagnosis. If necessary, recording devices that can be fitted to the patient so that an ambulatory ECG can be obtained are available.

(c) When the resting ECG is normal the next logical test is treadmill exercise testing. This is extremely sensitive, a positive result being obtained in approximately 90 per cent of patients. If positive, as the exercise period continues chest pain develops and ischaemic ST segment depression on the ECG appears. Such symptoms and signs, when the cardiac rate is still low, are highly suggestive of severe multivessel disease.

Treatment

Once the diagnosis has been confirmed attempts should be made to control the symptoms of the disease by—

1 control of diabetes if present;
2 avoidance or reversal of obesity;
3 trying to present hypercatecholaemia by the avoidance of smoking and, if possible, the avoidance of stress;
4 specific medication such as the use of the coronary vasodilator drug, glyceryl trinitrite.

The last-named drug is of proven value but the place of drugs intended either to control or reverse hyperlipidaemia is as yet unknown and the use of anticoagulant therapy appears to have little part to play in the long-term control of atherosclerosis.
Newer antiplatelet agents such as dipyridinol and pyridinol carbonate await evaluation.

Long-term outlook in patients suffering from coronary artery disease

One of the most important studies of this subject was made in the USA in Framingham, Massachusetts in a group of 5127 persons between the ages of 30 and 59 who were free of coronary artery disease. All these individuals were examined at two-year intervals and only an insignificant number were 'lost' during the following ten-year period. It was found—

1 that the overall ratio of men to women developing coronary heart disease, during the period of study was 2 : 1;
2 that the incidence of angina increased proportionally with advancing age, 6 males developing angina between 30 and 39 years of age and 37 in the period between 50 and 59;
3 the number of women developing angina rose rapidly and exceeded that of men in the sixth decade;
4 unexpectedly, however, the incidence of myocardial infarction increased much more steeply, 17 cases occurring in men in the fourth decade and 73 cases in the sixth decade, but whereas in patients complaining of angina the sex incidence became equal, with advancing age myocardial infarction was three times commoner in men than women in the sixth decade;
5 sudden death occurred almost exclusively in men rather than in women.

This data has been interpreted as meaning that while there is no great difference in the severity of coronary atherosclerosis in the two sexes there is a marked difference in the proneness to thrombosis.

Biochemical aspects

Among the many biochemical factors investigated the one that appeared to be of greatest importance was the cholesterol level; the higher the serum cholesterol the greater the risk of coronary artery disease.

Physiological aspects

Important in the physiological sense was the systolic blood pressure, the morbidity from coronary heart disease being appreciably greater the higher the systolic blood pressure.

Social factors

The most important of these were obesity and cigarette smoking. The effect of the former was to increase the incidence of angina and of the latter to increase the incidence of myocardial infarction.

Indications for coronary artery surgery

The most common indication for coronary artery bypass surgery is the development of angina pectoris uncontrolled by 'medical' regimes. The fundamental cause of such angina is the inability of the coronary circulation to supply the sudden increases in ventricular oxygen demand that occur during exercise or emotional stress. The result is a decrease in the ratio of coronary blood flow to tissue metabolism.

INVESTIGATIONS REQUIRED BEFORE CONSIDERING CORONARY ARTERY BYPASS SURGERY

Once it has been established that medical treatment is ineffective and that bypass surgery should be considered the following investigations must be performed.

1   Noninvasive radionuclide imaging

This technique, which was introduced in 1973, enables the myocardium to be visualised by the use of a rectilinear scanner following the injection of ^{43}K which has a half-life of 22 hours, or ^{201}Thalium with a half-life of 73 hours. A uniform pattern of myocardinal nuclide accumulation occurs in patients at rest or during exercise who are not suffering from coronary artery disease. Patients suffering from a previous transmural myocardial infarct will have regions of decreased accumulation corresponding to the electrocardiographic localisation of this damaged area. It is also possible to demonstrate by this technique areas of transient ischaemia.

2   Cardiac catheterisation

(a)   Technique

Although invasive, this technique permits the haemodynamic status of the myocardium to be established and by using selective coronary artery cineangiography it is also possible to delineate sequential coronary artery obstruction.

The catheters required can be introduced either via the brachial or the femoral arteries and they should be radio-opaque so that they can be radiographically visualised at frequent intervals.

(b)   Findings

Selective angiography usually demonstrates the site, extent, and severity of the pathological segment of the artery although there is still some disagreement as to the severity of narrowing required to produce a decrease in myocardial blood flow.

It has been shown that arterial stenosis that produces only 50 per cent luminal obstruction will compromise the blood flow only if a substantial length of the artery is involved. Much more significant are lesions causing stenosis of 75 per cent or more.

Distribution of atherosclerotic lesions

This has been repeatedly investigated by angiographic and autopsy studies. The worst affected vessel, and the one that is nearly always involved, is the anterior descending branch of the left coronary artery. Thereafter, in descending order of frequency of involvement are, the main right coronary vessel, 25 to 40 per cent; the left circumflex 5 to 33 per cent; the main left artery in 10 per cent and, finally, the posterior descending branch of the left artery.

In addition to these major lesions, in females especially, the smaller distal segments of the major vessels are frequently involved.

Various scoring techniques based on the radiological findings have been described in order to assess the severity of the arterial changes. While of little interest to the surgeon who has already decided on a surgical approach the results of such assessments are certainly significant when considering the eventual outcome of the disease, since patients with high scores tend to die as a result of myocardial infarction within five years of investigation.

Physiological investigations

In addition to the anatomical evidence cardiac angiography provides, a variety of measurements of cardiac function can also be obtained. One of the most important of these is the LVEDP (left ventricular end diastolic pressure) which is a measure of left ventricular function. Elevation of this value above 25 mmHg is associated with diffuse arterial disease, generalised myocardial degeneration, and early mortality following operation.

DIRECT CORONARY ARTERY BYPASS SURGERY

The insertion of the first saphenous vein aortocoronary bypass graft was performed in the Methodist Hospital, Houston, Texas, in 1964 but the operation did not gain more general acceptance until 1967. By 1974 it was estimated that some 100 000 operations of this type had been carried out in the United States alone and it has been estimated that in 1977 this number was performed in a single year.

The development of bypass surgery was preceded by an era in which attempts were made to increase the vascularity of the myocardium in a variety of indirect ways. Among these were—

(a)   the removal of the epicardium followed by omental grafting;
(b)   Vineberg's operation, in which the internal mammary artery was implanted into the myocardium.

The importance of these earlier operations lies not so much in the fact that they failed to improve the blood flow to the damaged myocardium but rather that they often produced a remarkable, if temporary, relief in the symptoms of which the patient complained, by presumably, a placebo effect.

Present status of bypass surgery

The status of coronary artery bypass surgery is still dubious to many. This is particularly so in that there is some evidence that the natural history of coronary artery disease is changing. This suggestion finds support from two entirely different sources—

(a) Insurance statistics of the USA, Australia, and Finland all show that the number of deaths from coronary artery disease is declining.

(b) Autopsy findings in members of the armed forces killed in two conflicts, in Korea and Vietnam, the two wars being separated by 15 years. In the former, 73 per cent of the victims had some degree of atheroma, in 15 per cent resulting in over 50 per cent narrowing in one or more coronary vessels, whereas in the latter only 45 per cent showed evidence of the disease and in only 5 per cent was it severe.

There is, however, little disagreement that bypass surgery produces a high incidence of symptomatic relief, particularly if the technique of sequential grafting is adopted to overcome a series of blocks, but there is no conclusive evidence that coronary artery surgery substantially reduces the risk of death from myocardial infarction in future years.

However, the argument centres on—

(a)   the reasons for the good results obtained;
(b)   the question of graft patency;
(c)   the dangers of subsequently developing a coronary thrombosis.

Various studies suggest that the initial results are not sustained and that as many as 12 per cent of patients relapse within 24 to 48 months following surgery. The mechanism of pain relief may not necessarily be due only to the increasing blood flow beyond the point of significant obstruction. In some patients it may be due to—

(a) denervation of the ischaemic areas resulting from the necessary dissection of the coronary vessels and epicardium;

(b) the development of a perioperative myocardial infarct, a suggestion made probable by the finding that Q waves, together with changes in serum enzyme levels occur in from 1 to 40 per cent of patients, depending on the series examined;

(c) a simple placebo effect, 60 per cent of patients subjected to Beck's operation, which is known to be anatomically ineffective, being rendered symptom free.

Graft patency

So far as graft patency is concerned the majority of reports indicate that one of the major factors determining this is the state of the distal vascular bed, but in nearly all series it has been reported that the intima of the venous graft rapidly thickens so that the demonstrable lumen is reduced by 30 to 50 per cent although overall graft patency remains high, over 80 per cent being patent at 6 years.

It has now been established that coronary bypass surgery should seldom be performed on patients who have suffered from a recent myocardial infarct because of the prohibitive mortality, which falls to reasonable levels only after about three months.

4.3 DEEP VEIN THROMBOSIS, DIAGNOSIS AND PROPHYLAXIS

Incidence. The precise incidence of deep venous thrombosis following surgical procedure is still debatable. Some of the various frequencies that have been quoted are—

(a) following comparative minor surgery such as inguinal herniorrhaphy, 26 per cent;
(b) following major surgery, 42 per cent;
(c) following 'strokes' of sufficient severity to produce immobilisation of a leg or after immobilisation following severe fractures, 60 per cent.

Aetiological factors

Virchow (1850) pronounced that the development of thromboembolic phenomena was dependent upon the following factors—

1 *Changes in the blood.* These involve both the quantitative and qualitative changes occurring in the platelets, particularly following operation, or in patients suffering from malignant disease. As regards the former, investigation has shown that increased platelet adhesiveness follows surgery, and specifically following splenectomy there is a considerable increase in the actual number of platelets in the circulation, the count rising from the normal range of between $150 - 400 \times 10^9$/litre to a height of over 900×10^9/litre at which level spontaneous thrombosis may occur. Following moderately severe surgery or injury without interference with the spleen the platelet count gradually rises during the first 10 to 14 days after which it returns to normal within three weeks.

In addition to changes in platelet number and adhesiveness there are also changes in the coagulation and fibrinolytic mechanisms, although the relative importance of each remains to be determined. According to one hypothesis a dynamic equilibrium exists between the clotting and lysis of blood. The latter depends upon the plasminogen system and following trauma or surgical interference the plasminogen activator activity increases, this material coming from the vein wall and tissue damaged at the time of surgery. It has also been shown that patients who have suffered a pulmonary embolus have a very low level of fibrinolytic activity.

2 *Changes in the characteristics of blood flow.* The velocity of the venous blood from the lower limbs undoubtedly decreases during surgery and in the immediate postoperative period when the patient is relatively immobilised. It is said, not without some truth, that the patient in greatest danger of developing a pulmonary embolus is the individual who has been moved from a medical to a surgical division following prolonged investigation. Partial obstruction followed by a reduction in the velocity of blood flow may well be the explanation of the development of calf thrombosis in an individual after a prolonged drive in a vehicle during which both the thigh and the knee are flexed to a right angle.

In some operations the blood flow from the lower limb may be almost brought to a halt; for example—

(*a*)   during hip arthroplasty when the hip is dislocated, the femoral vein resembles a 'cork-screw' and the blood flow from the leg and thigh virtually ceases.

(*b*)   during peripheral arterial surgery involving the lower limb when the common femoral artery is occluded during the performance of a vein graft or profundoplasty.

(*c*)   in severe trauma to the lower limb or pelvis.

3 *Changes in the vessel wall.* These are predominantly the result of endothelial damage to the calf veins by compression, particularly during the period of total relaxation on an unguarded operating table. However, in various groups deep venous thrombosis is more common than in others. These include patients suffering from multiple injuries, cardiac disease, the obese, the anaemic, the polycythaemic, the hemiplegic, and patients suffering from malignant disease.

Predictive methods

By analysis of the following variables, euglobulin lysis time, age, the presence of varicose veins, fibrin-related antigen, and percentage overweight, one group of investigators has shown that it is possible to identify 95 per cent of patients undergoing gynaecological operations who will develop a deep venous thrombosis, misallocating only about a third. Of the changes described, the laboratory factor with the greatest predictive power was the euglobulin lysis time, which measures the time taken for lysis of the euglobulin fraction of the plasma. After this the age of the patient assumed greatest significance.

If the results of such predictive methods are confirmed they will be of considerable value because they will reduce the number of individuals who may be given, and therefore may suffer, the possible complications of anticoagulant therapy.

Diagnosis

The recognition of deep vein thrombosis was, in the past, an entirely clinical exercise. The important symptom is a complaint of pain in the calf, usually on or about the fifth postoperative day which is associated with muscular tenderness and may or may not be associated with swelling. If this is minimal it involves only the foot and ankle, but severe and extensive venous involvement produces the syndromes of phlegmasia alba dolens (the large white leg) or phlegmasia caerulea dolens (the large blue leg). The importance of the latter syndrome is that it is nearly always associated with some loss of tissue. Fortunately, this commonly involves the toe pads only.

METHODS OF INVESTIGATION

1 Ultrasonography

The advantage of ultrasonography is that it is noninvasive. The two disadvantages are that it is impossible by this method to detect nonocclusive disease in the major veins, or detect the presence of thrombosis restricted to the calf veins.

When using ultrasonography, a Doppler probe is placed on the groin, and when the sounds of the femoral artery are identified the probe is moved some millimetres medially over the femoral vein. The Doppler signals from a patent vein consist of a continuous rushing noise. Sudden compression of a normal limb produces a distinct brief and high-pitched noise called the 'augmented flow sound'. Absence indicates occlusion. Alternatively, fluctuations in proximal flow can be induced by asking the patient to perform a Valsalva manoeuvre. Obviously, in the presence of severe proximal occlusion no change in flow can occur.

2 Plethysmography

This method has also been adopted, using, in particular, changes in electrical impedance in the limb due to the presence of thrombi. Although evaluated this method remains predominantly of research interest.

3   Isotopic methods

The chief method available for the diagnosis of calf vein thrombosis is the injection of ^{125}I labelled fibrinogen. The procedure however, is, relatively time consuming. The isotopically labelled fibrinogen must be injected immediately following the operation, and thereafter the emission rate is counted over a number of fixed points in the legs and thighs daily, using the praecordial count as the control. Any sudden increase in the count over a particular area is regarded as the probable site of intravascular thrombosis since, in the presence of a clot, the radioactive fibrinogen is incorporated into it, thus producing the 'hot' spot. The count is regarded as significant only when it rises by at least 15 per cent, and the elevation should persist and even increase in both magnitude and extent on succeeding days.

Investigations using this technique have shown that venous thrombosis is twice as common as might be expected from the results of an ordinary clinical examination and can be expected in about 25 per cent of middle-aged or elderly patients undergoing surgery. The method is particularly valuable for the diagnosis of calf vein thrombosis, but its accuracy decreases as the inguinal ligament is approached and it cannot be used for the diagnosis of thrombosis in the common femoral or iliac vein. It compares in accuracy with venography (*see* below) and counts can be made for up to 7 days before decay makes the isotope too difficult to identify. Prior to its use, however, the pateint should be tested for iodine sensitivity, and uptake of iodine by the thyroid should be blocked by daily administration of iodine; 150 mg of sodium iodide. This method is obviously invalidated in the presence of a haematoma and is, therefore, useless after lower limb arterial surgery.

4   Venography

This technique was first described by Dos Santos and popularised by Bauer. The radio-opaque contrast medium is injected into the veins on the dorsum of the foot and is directed into the deep system by the use of ankle torniquets. Alternatively, the medium can be injected directly into the deep venous system by a needle placed into the calcaneum. The latter method is seldom used, however, because of the potential danger of osteomyelitis in the bone.

Progress of the medium along the veins is followed by screening and appropriately delayed radiographs. Unfortunately, phlebography is of little use for demonstrating clot in the sinusoids of the calf muscles, and it is a time-consuming investigation that cannot be regarded as a routine diagnostic procedure.

Thrombus or clot produces well-defined filling defects in the venous channels. Loose clot appears as a cylindrical or rounded translucent defect separated from the vein wall by a fine white line of contrast medium. Absence of this line indicates adherence of the clot to the intimal layer of the vein, a process usually complete within four days of its formation.

Confusion may be caused by underfilling of the veins, dilution of the contrast medium on reaching the relatively larger veins from the smaller tributaries, and the stream-lining of the contrast medium.

PROPHYLAXIS

The methods of prophylaxis that have been used to prevent deep venous thrombosis include—

1 medical methods designed to alter the coagulability of the blood;
2 physical methods designed to maintain lower limb venous blood flow during surgery.

Medical methods

This method requires the administration of either heparin or dextran 70.

(*a*) *Heparin*. This drug acts towards the end stage of the clotting mechanism by inhibiting the conversion of fibrinogen to fibrin. It is a direct anticoagulant and inhibits clotting both in vitro and in vivo but it will not produce lysis in vitro. Its use is contra-indicated in patients suffering from bleeding disorders or ulceration of the gastrointestinal tract.

Used prophylactically to prevent the development of deep venous thrombosis a variety of different regimes have been suggested, among which are—

(i) Subcutaneous injection of 5000 IU 2 hours before surgery, 24 hours after surgery and then every 12 hours for five days.
(ii) 5000 IU 2 hours before surgery and then two doses at 12-hourly intervals.

Other but similar regimes described have been shown to lower the incidence of thrombosis from levels as high as 42 per cent in controls, to between 4 and 10 per cent in the patients receiving heparin.

(*b*) *Dextran 70*. Dextrans are produced by the fermentation of sucrose by Leuconostoc mesenteroides. It has been suggested that in order to prevent deep vein thrombosis an infusion of dextran 70 should be started immediately before the induction of anaesthesia, and continued for six hours. The beneficial effect of dextran is due to the reduction in platelet adhesiveness that follows its administration so that there is minimal aggregation of these elements following injury which, in turn, reduces the amount of thrombokinase present and eliminates the end-stage clotting mechanism.

Other drugs that have been suggested include aspirin in a dose of 800 mg daily. The early extremely satisfactory results obtained by this method do not appear to have been substantiated, however, in later trials.

Comparison of heparin and dextran

In one, large randomised trial the efficacy of heparin was compared with that of dextran 70 and both were compared with a control group receiving no treatment. Heparin was given in a dose of 2500 units subcutaneously two hours before operation followed by 5000 units twice daily until the seventh postoperative day. Three 500 ml infusions of dextran 70 were given, the first at operation and the second and third on the first and second postoperative days. The ^{125}I fibrinogen test was used to detect calf thrombosis, and the following results were obtained: venous thrombosis occurred in 37 per cent of the controls, 25 per cent of the patients receiving dextran 70, and only 12 per cent of those receiving heparin, suggesting therefore, that the latter was the significantly better method of prophylaxis.

Disadvantages of medical control

The protection afforded by either heparin or dextran 70 may cause increasing technical difficulties because of oozing, which may, if continuing into the postoperative period, lead to haematoma formation.

Significance of a deep venous thrombosis

The true significance of subclinical thrombosis in the calf veins remains to be established although there is some evidence that proximal spread subsequently occurs in about one-third of patients, and there can be little doubt this increases the danger of pulmonary embolism. For example, in one reported trial involving over 800 patients treated either by saline injections alone or by two infusions of 500 ml of dextran it was found that the incidence of calf vein thrombosis was similar in the two groups but that the incidence of pulmonary embolism was greatly reduced in the dextran treated group. The conclusion reached was, therefore, that calf vein thrombosis was of little clinical significance except in relation to main vein thrombosis involving the ileofemoral segments.

Physical methods of prophylaxis

A variety of physical methods designed to maintain the venous circulation during surgery have been described. These include—
   (*a*) The mechanical pumping of the venous blood from the legs by the use of—

   (i)   inflatable plastic leggings;
   (ii) intermittent electrical stimulation of the calf muscles;
   (iii) pedal treadmills operating throughout the period of operation.

(b) The use of elastic stockings that produce different pressures on various parts of the lower limb and that may be worn both during the operation and throughout the early postoperative period.

The advantage of physical methods over medical methods lies in the absence of any changes in the blood itself, hence there is no increase in the technical difficulties associated with surgery.

4.4 THE COMPLICATIONS OF VENOUS THROMBOSIS, DIAGNOSIS AND TREATMENT

The major complications that follow deep venous thrombosis are the immediate development of thromboembolic phenomena and the late development of varicose ulceration. The latter is discussed in *Tutorials in Surgery I.*

Most emboli are silent, causing neither complaint nor observable physical signs; indeed, only 30 per cent of patients have the classic triad of tender calves, pleural pain, and haemoptysis, although sudden collapse followed by death occurs in approximately 20 per cent. Classically, this event occurs while straining at stool. Overall, between 3 and 5 per cent of hospital deaths are caused by pulmonary thromboembolism. A pulmonary embolus should, however, be suspected in any patient, whatever age, who about the tenth postoperative day develops chest pain, tachypnoea or mild cyanosis.

Physical examination in such patients may reveal such physical signs as decreased breath sounds, râles, rhonchi and/or a pleural rub. Blood may be noted in the sputum.

INVESTIGATION

Plain X-ray of chest

(a)   This may appear normal even when there has been a massive pulmonary embolus involving at least 50 per cent of the vascular tree, although careful inspection may reveal hyperlucent areas caused by a paucity of vascular filling and indicating pulmonary oligaemia. The main pulmonary artery may be enlarged and the hilar shadows may appear plump. Should the patient survive, the increase in girth of the hilum rapidly disappears as the clot undergoes lysis and fragmentation.

(b)   Infarction following obstruction to the lobar or segmental arteries occurs only in about 15 per cent of patients because of the dual blood supply to the lungs from pulmonary and bronchial vessels, but when it does occur a pulmonary opacity develops. This is most commonly seen in the lower lobes, it often lies adjacent to one or two pleural surfaces, and it is frequently associated with elevation of the diaphragm on the affected side.

The classic configuration of the pulmonary shadow is that of a homogenous wedge-shaped area of variable size in the peripheral lung fields, with the base contiguous to a visceral pleural surface, and an apex, often rounded, directed towards the hilum, the so-called Hampton's Hump. If the infarct involves a whole lobe, resolution may take several weeks and the patient may remain ill, suffering from pulmonary symptoms such as dyspnoea and a pyrexia which is totally unaffected by antibiotics.

(c)   Commoner than the 'typical infarct' are line shadows in the lung fields and these may take various forms. Usually, they are linear areas of increased density which form horizontal shadows in the lower lobes. Serial X-rays frequently show that these opaque zones become increasingly linear with the passage of time. In addition to the parenchymal changes pleural effusions are common if the infarct is of any size.

2   Pulmonary angiography

This is performed by introducing a catheter via the antecubital vein until its tip lies in the main pulmonary artery, after which a suitable radio-opaque dye is injected. An embolus is normally seen as a filling defect within the artery but this investigation is of little value if the embolus has fragmented and so gained access to vessels of 2 mm or less in diameter. An advantage pulmonary angiography possesses over lung scanning is the ease with which filling defects in the lower lobes, in which postoperative emboli are nearly always situated, can be identified, this being the area least effectively visualised by radioisotope scanning.

3   Lung scan

This is performed by injecting macroaggregates of albumin tagged with labelled iodine, chromium, or technetium. These macroaggregates are two to five times the size of erythrocytes and are, therefore, capable of blocking the lung capillaries. They are, however, easily fragmented and therefore produce only temporary occlusion. Four standard projections of the chest are normally taken, posterior, anterior, and right and left lateral. The posterior view is regarded as the most important since it encompasses the greatest volume of lung.

A positive scan, indicating the presence of a pulmonary embolus, reveals areas of diminished perfusion in the affected lung field. These follow a segmental distribution and usually extend to the periphery of the lung and sometimes possess the shape of a truncated cone. Several defects are usually present since even a single large embolus soon fragments and is, therefore, able to make its way into the more peripheral vessels.

4 Electrocardiography

The changes, if any, seen on the electrocardiogram are determined by—

(a) the size of the embolus;
(b) the interval between embolisation and the performance of the investigation.

The classical changes, highly suggestive of an acute embolus, are—

(a) the appearance of an S wave on Lead I;
(b) an inverted Q wave or T wave or both in Lead III.

Less reliable are those changes indicating right axis deviation, possibly right bundle branch block or right ventricular hypertrophy.

5 Biochemical tests

Cellular enzyme studies may be of value. After a recent pulmonary embolus the concentration of lactic dehydrogenase (LDH) may be raised well above its normal level of 90 to 350 IU/litre. Unfortunately, a similar elevation may also occur following a myocardial infarction, but in this condition another enzyme unaffected by a pulmonary embolus, aspartate aminotransferase (AST), is also elevated above its normal value to 10 to 50 IU/litre. Should either condition, therefore, be suspected the level of both enzymes should be estimated as one may be clinically indistinguishable from the other.

TREATMENT OF PULMONARY EMBOLUS

1 Medical

(a) Heparin and Warfarin

The most common treatment for any patient who suffers from a pulmonary embolus is the institution of properly controlled anticoagulant therapy. This is done to prevent the further extension of clot and so diminish the chances of a repeated embolus. Suggested regimes for the use of heparin consist of the administration of 10 000 units four-hourly for 24 hours, then six-hourly or, alternatively, a continuous intravenous heparin drip, administering 40 000 units in the first 24 hours and thereafter, 20 000 units daily. Haemorrhage, if it should occur, is treated by the antidote Protamine sulphate BP slowly injected intravenously in a dose of 1 mg for every 100 units of heparin last used.

If the patient has suffered a pulmonary embolus anticoagulant therapy is normally continued for several weeks. It is, therefore, customary to begin the administration of one of the indirect anticoagulants after 48 hours, the two in common use being Phenindione BP (Dindevan) and Warfarin BP.

The normal loading dose of Phenindione is 200 to 300 mg which should produce a therapeutic prothrombin time of 30 within 18 to 24 hours. The continuation dose lies between 25 and 100 mg daily in divided doses and is judged by monitoring the prothrombin time. If there has been an over-dosage and immediate reversal is required, Phytomenadione BP, which is a naturally occurring Vitamin K, is administered orally or intravenously in a dose of between 5 and 20 mg.

The initial dose of Warfarin is 50 mg and a therapeutic effect can be expected within 12 to 18 hours.

There is no well-documented account as to how long antiocoagulant therapy should be continued but as a rule a period of three months should probably be allowed to elapse before ceasing treatment. This allows adequate time for the clot to become organised, recanalised, and covered with endothelium.

(b) Streptokinase

An alternative method of treating either an established progressive thrombus or a pulmonary embolus is by the use of the drug streptokinase, a substance obtained from culture filtrates of the β-haemolytic streptococcus belonging to Lancefield Group C. The mechanism of action is activation of the intrinsic fibrinolytic system by the formation of a linkage compound between the drug itself and the pro-activator plasminogen molecule. This complex brings about the conversion of plasminogen into the fibrinolytic enzyme plasmin which lyses thrombi that are mainly fibrinoid in character; its effect on the platelet-rich white thrombi being much less evident.

Streptokinase is given by intravascular infusion, the initial dose over a period of 30 min, after which the maintenance dose is continued by slow infusion by means of a mechanical pump. The standard initial dose, which is entirely arbitrary is 250 000 IU. This priming dose is then followed by a maintenance dose of 100 000 IU hourly until clinical improvement is observed. The various reports in the literature devoted to this subject show that considerable success can be achieved but recurrence of thrombosis despite the simultaneous administration of anticoagulants appears to be relatively common.

Should serious haemorrhage occur in the course of treatment administration of streptokinase should stop and an intravenous infusion of 20 to 50 ml of 10 per cent epsilonaminocaproic acid started. This displaces the streptokinase from the activator molecule and reverses its effect. Streptokinase is antigenic, and it is therefore advisable to cover the first dose by a single 100 mg dose of hydrocortisone hemisuccinate and avoid all further use of the drug for a period of some three months.

Apart from inducing haemorrhage, either from the operation site or from some coincidental condition such as gastroduodenal ulceration, some patients develop rigors following treatment.

(c) Ancrod therapy

Ancrod is a proteolytic enzyme derived from the fractionation of the venom of the Malayan pit viper. If bitten by such a snake over a third of the victims show a prolonged haemostatic defect. This observation has led to its limited clinical use as an anticoagulant, especially in patients suffering from severe ileofemoral thrombosis or established pulmonary embolus. Its effectiveness, however, does not appear to be as great as the forms of therapy described above.

2 Surgical

In some patients the treatment of massive ileofemoral thrombosis or recurrent pulmonary emboli by means of anticoagulants may be contra-indicated. Such patients include those known to be suffering from peptic ulceration, a bleeding tendency, recent cerebrovascular accident, or hepatic failure.

In this group resort has been made to mechanical interruption of the inferior vena cava, a method first adopted by Trendelenberg in 1917 when he ligated the inferior vena cava in a patient suffering from suppurative pelvic thrombophlebitis.

(A) Caval interruption

The methods adopted to achieve this include—

(a) *Ligation.* This was the first and, according to many surgeons, remains the best method of preventing recurrent emboli. The cava is blocked by a ligature placed just below the renal veins, a level at which it is considered that:

(i) the occlusion will be above any thrombus;
(ii) the flow from the renal veins will prevent thrombosis in the cava proximal to the ligature.

The opponents of this method claim that it carries a high incidence of undesirable sequelae. Of these the most immediate is the profound fall in venous return to the heart which compromises the cardiac output and causes the blood pressure to fall.

In a large series of 119 cases it has been clearly shown that preoperative cardiac function governs the outcome of caval ligation and that this form of treatment is contra-indicated in the presence of heart failure. Later, the consequences of stasis become important. Such is the conflicting evidence in the literature that it is impossible to give a precise opinion as to the importance of this, especially as any such sequelae must be partly due to the postphlebitic syndrome following the actual venous thrombosis rather than the caval interruption. However, it has been clearly demonstrated that bilateral venous stasis occurs in patients in whom only a unilateral thrombosis was initially present.

(b) *Plication.* This procedure, first described by Spencer in 1962, requires the mobilisation of 3 to 4 cm of the cava and the insertion of between 3 and 5 sutures across its lumen, making channels 3 to 4-mm wide. The high patency rate of the cava following this operation reduces the incidence of postoperative stasis.

(c) *Clipping.* This may be performed using a smooth or serrated Teflon clip, either variety being relatively easy to insert if the cava has been adequately mobilised.

(d) *The Mobin-Uddin intracaval umbrella introduced in 1969.* This device resembles an umbrella with stainless-steel spokes between which are heparinised silastic panels that may be perforated or unperforated. The umbrella is inserted in a folded position into the internal jugular vein under local anaesthesia. Under direct radiological vision it is then passed down into the inferior vena cava to a position just inferior to the renal veins. These are previously indirectly located from the position of the renal pelves which have themselves been indirectly located at the time of pulmonary angiography. Once at the correct level the umbrella is opened, and by slight upward traction on the guide wire the small projections of the spokes beyond the panels fix the device in position, after which the guide wire is unscrewed and removed. The main advantage of this technique is that it can be used in high-risk patients. However, the heart action should be continuously monitored by ECG as cardiac irregularities tend to occur as the device passes through the right atrium.

(B) *Pulmonary embolectomy*

This operation was first advocated in 1908 by Trendelenberg. However, approximately 95 per cent of patients who suffer a massive immediately occlusive embolus usually die before any operative steps can be taken to save them. However, the remaining patients survive for periods of up to an hour and it is in this group that, with the introduction of cardio-pulmonary bypass, the operation instead of being performed in haste can be performed in a leisurely fashion, the peripheral emboli being removed by suction.

4.5 VASCULAR LESIONS OF THE INTESTINAL TRACT AND THEIR CONSEQUENCES

ANATOMY OF THE INTESTINAL CIRCULATION

Arterial

The stomach and duodenum are supplied by branches of the coeliac axis artery; the small intestine and proximal part of the colon by the superior mesenteric artery; the distal colon from the junction of the middle and lateral thirds of the transverse colon by the inferior mesenteric arteries; and the rectum by the middle and inferior haemorrhoidal arteries.

Superior mesenteric artery

The superior mesenteric artery, which is virtually an end artery, arises from the aorta at a level between the first and second lumbar vertebrae. Of the three major arteries arising from the abdominal aorta, its width and acute angle of origin make it the most likely blood vessel to catch an embolus. In its first few centimetres it lies behind the pancreas surrounded by a plexus of autonomic nerve ganglia and fibres, together with the tributaries of the portal vein. These anatomical relationships make the surgical approach to its origin a matter of considerable technical difficulty. Its first branch, the inferior pancreatico-duodenal artery, although small may form a significant collateral circulation with the superior pancreatico-duodenal artery which is a branch of the gastroduodenal artery which, in turn, is derived from the hepatic artery.

As the superior mesenteric artery passes downwards it crosses the anterior surface of the horizontal part of the duodenum, and because of this it may at times, particularly in patients who have lost a considerable amount of weight, usually as the result of operation or injury, become a significant cause of early postoperative obstruction, producing the condition known in the UK as duodenal ileus and, in the United States, the superior mesenteric artery syndrome.

As the superior mesenteric artery continues downwards within the mesentery of the small bowel it gives off from its left-hand side between 6 and 12 intestinal arteries which divide and reunite within the mesentery to form a series of arterial arcades. These become increasingly complex as the terminal ileum is approached, and from them, straight branches known as the vasa recti, run to alternating sides of the bowel wall. From the right-hand side of the main vessel the colic vessels, usually three in number, arise. These named vessels are known respectively as the middle colic, right colic, and ileocolic arteries. Unlike the intestinal vessels they do not form a complex arcade system, although all three are united by a marginal artery which runs along the mesentery in close proximity to the wall of the bowel. The result is that the ascending and transverse parts of the colon are much more vulnerable to injury or occlusion. In the region of the caecum the ileocolic artery anastomoses with the termination of the superior mesenteric.

Inferior mesenteric artery

The inferior mesenteric artery arises approximately 3 cm above the aortic bifurcation and supplies the colon from the splenic flexure to the junction of the upper and middle thirds of the rectum. The first branch of this artery, known as the upper left colic, meets the marginal vessel that arises from the middle colic artery in the region of the splenic flexure in an anastomosis which is often deficient, thus accounting for the frequency with which ischaemic changes are found in this area. The inferior mesenteric artery terminates in the superior haemorrhoidal artery which anastomoses within the rectal wall with branches of the middle rectal artery arising from the internal iliac artery.

Vasa Recti

The vasa recti enter the intestinal wall in a diagonal direction reaching, as previously described, alternate aspects of its wall. Each terminal artery supplies only 1 to 2 cm of bowel and it is not until the vessels have reached the submucous layer of the bowel wall that a rich submucous plexus is formed in which numerous arteriovenous shunts are found, particularly in the stomach and large bowel. Arterioles supply the villi, running up their centre close to the venule, and end in a network of capillaries.

The lack of anastomoses between the vasa recti potentially predisposes to a serious compromise of the blood supply to the antimesenteric border of the intestine during small bowel resection, and it is to ensure an adequate blood supply to this part of the intestinal wall that it is customary and necessary to transect the small intestine obliquely rather than at a right angle.

Venous Drainage

The venous drainage of the small intestine and colon is through tributaries of the inferior and superior mesenteric veins which ultimately drain into the portal vein. The venous drainage parallels the arterial supply except that the main trunk of the inferior mesenteric vein does not accompany the artery but rather courses upwards, lateral to the duodeno-jejunal flexure and a little lateral to the ligament of Treitz, and passing over the body of the pancreas joins with the splenic vein. A further point of clinical importance is the communication made between the inferior mesenteric vein carrying portal blood and the middle and inferior haemorrhoidal veins carrying systemic blood.

PHYSIOLOGY OF INTESTINAL CIRCULATION

The mesenteric circulation is controlled by both central and peripheral factors—

(a) Central factors include cardiac output and autonomic 'tone'. Mesenteric flow is reduced by any reduction in cardiac output which probably accounts for the numerous cases of non-occlusive necrosis associated with cardiac failure.

(b) The autonomic system affects both the arterioles and the musculature of the gut but the overall effect is far from clear. The gut has no baroreceptors and thus no protection against vasomotor reflexes which act at the expense of the mesenteric flow.

(c) Peripheral factors affecting the flow of blood to the bowel are a function of the vascular anatomy. The autoregulatory mechanisms can be impeded by a high venous pressure since the portal system is valveless and allows pressure in the intestinal veins to increase in the presence of portal obstruction.

PATHOLOGY OF VASCULAR OBSTRUCTION

Regardless of the cause of an arterial occlusion the effect is always to produce haemorrhagic necrosis of the bowel wall which has both characteristic macroscopic and microscopic features.

Since the mucosa is the part most sensitive to anoxia it is the first to be affected. Necrosis beginning in the mucosa then spreads rapidly through the thickness of the bowel wall to involve, finally, the muscularis propria. Once this layer is necrotic, perforation is virtually inevitable and peritonitis follows.

The classical external signs of impending bowel necrosis, seen most commonly at operations for the relief of either external or internal strangulation are—

(a) Engorgement and swelling of the bowel wall. In sudden complete arterial occlusion, this stage is preceded by intense vasospasm, together with spasm of the bowel wall, but this stage is rarely seen by the practising surgeon since it normally passes off within one to two hours.

(b) Loss of contractility.

(c) 'Bogginess' of the gut wall due to extravasation of blood into the wall of the gut and venous thrombosis.

(d) Cyanosis. This change in the colour rapidly progresses to a plum colour and, finally, a greenish-black discoloration of the affected segment.

(e) Loss of the peritoneal sheen and the exudation of serosanguineous fluid into the peritoneal cavity.

Depending on the cause of the occlusion these changes may terminate abruptly, as in the constriction rings of a strangulated internal or external hernia, or they may end somewhat less abruptly, particularly in the region of the duodeno-jejunal flexure, as in acute mesenteric thrombosis.

271

Should the patient survive an ischaemic attack, repair comes about by the formation of granulation tissue and, later, fibrosis. The constriction rings at each end of a strangulated loop may so fibrose and contract that eventually they cause intestinal obstruction, the intestinal stenosis of Garré, a rare but well-organised late complication that follows the relief of a strangulated internal or reduction of an external hernia.

Whatever the cause of intestinal ischaemia the ultimate fate of the bowel depends upon its duration. The gut is a unique organ, containing as it does within its lumen potentially destructive enzymes and pathogenic bacteria. When the gut becomes ischaemic bacteria invade its wall and toxins, notably endotoxins, are absorbed, producing not only an increase in the local inflammatory reaction within the wall of the bowel but also systemic effects in the form of endotoxaemic shock. In addition, because of the large surface area, estimated to be between 20 and 40 m^2 the massive exudation of fluid from the mucosa, which occurs following venous obstruction, is rapidly followed by hypovolaemic shock.

AETIOLOGY OF VASCULAR LESIONS

Congenital mesenteric vascular accidents

(a) Atresia

The cause of intestinal atresia remains uncertain. However, Louw of South Africa, produced a great deal of experimental evidence supporting the vascular theory of origin of this condition initially put forward by Jaboulay. The essence of Louw's work, which was performed on unborn dogs, was the demonstration that interruption of the vascular arcades of the small bowel mesentery in utero produces atresia, the severity of which is dependent upon the precise site of the vascular lesion. This theory gains support from the known embryological fact that the mesenteric circulation is in a state of 'flux' until the stage of rotation has been completed and also by the fact that exomphalos is commonly complicated by atresia.

(b) Volvulus

In the presence of malrotation and imperfect adhesion of the rotated bowel to the posterior abdominal wall a complete volvulus of the small bowel can occur around the axis of the superior mesenteric artery. The neonate presents in the manner typical of small bowel obstruction (*see Tutorials in Surgery I*, page 241) but this condition can be distinguished from simple obstruction by the rapidly deteriorating condition of the infant and the rapid development of oedema of the abdominal wall once ischaemia has developed.

Acquired arterial lesions

Acute bowel ischaemia in the adult may be caused by—

1 Obstruction of the blood supply by external compression of the mesentery. This occurs in:

(a) strangulated external herniae;
(b) strangulated internal herniae;
(c) volvulus;
(d) strangulation by congenital or acquired bands.

2 Thrombosis of a major blood vessel, usually occurring at the origin of the main arteries due to pre-existing atherosclerosis.

3 Embolus.

4 Involvement of the major arteries in aneurysmal dilatation.

5 Division or avulsion of the arterial supply following open or blunt injuries of the abdomen.

6 A low flow state, particularly if the mesenteric vessels are already the site of atherosclerosis. Such a condition may follow hypovolaemic hypotension, dehydration or the use of vasopressor agents. The patients at risk, therefore, are those who have sustained a recent myocardial infarction, who suffer from congestive heart failure or aortic incompetence, or cardiac arrhythmias, or who have developed hypovolaemia from any cause. The incidence of low flow nonocclusive mesenteric ischaemia has been estimated by various observers to be between 15 to 20 per cent of the whole.

ACUTE SUPERIOR MESENTERIC OCCLUSION AT ITS ORIGIN

Acute occlusion of the superior mesenteric artery usually occurs at its origin from the aorta or close to the origin of its middle colic branch, and it is more commonly due to embolism than thrombosis. Certain anatomical characteristics make the superior artery more susceptible to embolic occlusion than the inferior, the major factor being that the former leaves the aorta at an acute angle. The majority of emboli arise from the heart, either from a mural thrombosis following coronary thrombosis or an auricular thrombus developing in a fibrillating heart, but occasionally an embolus follows endocarditis, the spontaneous dislodgement of an atheromatous plaque from the aorta, or the accidental dislodgement of a plaque during translumbar aortography.

Thrombosis, which is less common, is always superimposed upon a vessel affected by atherosclerosis, the final event being frequently preceded by a period of hypotension.

Acute occlusion of the superior mesenteric artery or its branches always leads to gangrene of a variable length of the small intestine, depending on the site of the occlusion. Acute occlusion of the inferior mesenteric artery, however, is usually well tolerated provided the occlusion is limited to the origin of the vessel, the superior mesenteric artery is patent, and the collateral circulation is intact. It may, for example, have been interrupted by a previous bowel resection.

273

Clinical presentation of total superior mesenteric occlusion

The sudden onset of generalised abdominal pain in a male between 50 to 60 years of age, initially colicky but later becoming constant, is highly suggestive of mesenteric arterial occlusion, particularly if the individual suffers from cardiac disease. Initially, physical examination reveals generalised tenderness, but if the condition goes unrecognised rigidity develops and the bowel sounds disappear, usually within 12 hours.

Investigations

1 Plain X-ray of the abdomen. This at first shows no abnormality but as infarction develops, followed by ileus, multiple fluid levels appear.

2 Haematological investigations reveal a raised haematocrit and an elevated white cell count.

3 Biochemical investigation may reveal an elevated blood urea due to extravascular fluid loss and some elevation in the serum amylase, a finding that may make the distinction between vascular occlusion and acute pancreatitis difficult.

4 In some centres, if the diagnosis is suspected an abdominal angiogram is performed. Assuming the diagnosis is confirmed, an operation appropriate to the aetiology of the condition is undertaken. It has also been suggested that use should be made of the arterial catheter to administer an intravascular injection of papaverine.

Surgical Treatment

(a) Before infarction

The various surgical manoeuvres that have been suggested when the cause is thrombosis within an atherosclerotic vessel if laparotomy is performed prior to infarction, include endarterectomy, by-pass vein graft, or re-implanation of the superior mesentery artery. At the time that any of these operations is performed consequental clot should be removed by means of a Fogarty catheter, and if the superior mesenteric artery is opened it should be closed with a vein patch.

When the cause is arterial embolisation, embolectomy alone is required by means of a Fogarty catheter.

(b) Following infarction

The only possible treatment is surgical resection. In cases of occlusion of the superior mesenteric artery at its origin this normally entails a resection extending from a point just distal to duodeno-jejunal flexure to the junction of the transverse colon with the splenic flexure. Because of the severe metabolic consequences of such a procedure it has been suggested that doubtful areas should be left in situ and that the abdomen should be re-opened 24 hours later when the state of the remaining bowel can be reassessed. The author has had the opportunity of pursuing this policy in only one case.

Mortality

The mortality of acute occlusion when infarction has already occurred is high, and is variously reported as between 70 to 90 per cent. Survival, if operation is undertaken prior to infarction, may be as high as 50 per cent, but such survival figures can only be obtained in the presence of a high level of clinical suspicion. Note the axiom of Bacue and Austin that abdominal pain in a cardiac patient is embolic obstruction until proved otherwise.

INFERIOR MESENTERIC ARTERY OCCLUSION

1 Sudden occlusion of the inferior mesenteric artery may be the result of—

(*a*)   atheromatous involvement;
(*b*)   aortic aneurysm;
(*c*)   dissecting aneurysm of the aorta;
(*d*)   mesenteric haematoma;
(*e*)   thromboangitis obliterans.

Normally, the inferior mesenteric artery can be ligated at any point without interfering with bowel function because of the extensive collateral circulation through the anastomoses that exist between its branches, the middle colic and haemorrhoidal vessels. The former, a branch of the superior mesenteric artery, and the latter, the middle haemorrhoidal arteries. When infarction occurs there is nearly always impairment of this collateral network, usually due to co-existent atheroma in other vessels or previous surgical division following colonic resection.

2 Non-occlusive causes of large bowel circulatory disturbance include diabetes mellitus which particularly affects small vessels, rheumatoid arthritis, collagen diseases, embolic phenomena, disseminated intra-vascular coagulation, hypovolaemia, and cardiac failure.

ISCHAEMIC COLITIS

Up to 1966, when Marston and others published their classical paper on ischaemic colitis, only infrequent reports of disease of the large bowel, based on deprivation of arterial blood, had been reported. As had been previously observed, if the length of the bowel deprived of its blood supply is greater than the marginal and intramural vessels can supply, then necrosis, sloughing, and death from peritonitis is inevitable. However, as Marston pointed out, a situation can occur in which just enough blood reaches the bowel to prevent complete death of the intestine but at the same time is insufficient to sustain the mucosa. Necrosis of the latter follows and is accompanied by bacterial invasion.

The end result is again determined by the length of bowel involved. Should this be limited and an adequate collateral circulation exists the period of transient ischaemia may be followed by total resolution. Should the length of bowel be longer, and the collateral circulation ineffective, the end result, assuming that gangrene and perforation do not occur, may well be the development of a fibrous stricture most commonly in the region of the splenic flexure or descending colon.

Clinical Presentation

The clinical features of this condition are the sudden onset of lower abdominal pain, in an elderly patient, accompanied by vomiting and fever. Many patients pass either bright red blood or clots per rectum and in the majority there is no previous history of bowel disturbance, suggesting the presence of idiopathic colitis or Crohn's disease. However, in some patients a history of previous minor episodes may be elicited.

Should the condition proceed to gangrene, there is usually evidence of peritonitis within 12 hours, and examination of the abdomen shows rigidity and rebound tenderness, together with absent bowel sounds. An important physical sign that helps to distinguish this syndrome from *perforated* diverticulitis is the presence of blood either fresh or dark on the finger-stall following rectal examination.

When gangrene is averted, the patient may present with a much longer history and one suggesting the presence of idiopathic ulcerative colitis or colonic Crohn's disease. Such a history would include generalised malaise, intermittent abdominal pain, and diarrhoea. Should the lesion be extensive, sigmoidoscopy may reveal the presence of an abnormal mucosa with free bleeding. Plain X-ray of the abdomen may be negative or reveal a picture similar to toxic megacolon.

In some patients the ischaemic attack may be transient, leading to the syndrome sometimes known as evanescent colitis in which the patient presents in a symptomless state having suffered in the recent past an attack of left-sided abdominal pain and bloody motions.

Contrast Radiology

Contrast radiology of the colon may be normal if an attack of transient ischaemia has occurred; otherwise it may show stricture formation, usually involving the splenic flexure, together with changes of variable length in the transverse and descending colon.

The abnormalities related to the strictured area include 'thumb-printing', in which a polypoid-like change occurs and causes the appearance of a scalloped margin to the bowel wall with translucent, rounded, filling defects extending into the lumen in the filled phase of the barium enema, and showing as soft tissue masses in double contrast films. Ragged 'saw toothed' irregularity, tubular narrowing and sacculation may be seen. The last-named consist of shallow wide-mouthed outpouchings or pseudo-diverticula of the colonic wall.

The value of aortography, a potentially dangerous invasive technique, is doubtful but in some series it has been an 'occasional' investigation and the demonstration of occluded colic vessels has been reported.

Treatment

1 *In the presence of signs of peritonitis*

Laparotomy is indicated, followed by resection of the gangrenous bowel and, possibly, both a proximal and distal colostomy. If the general condition of the patient is satisfactory an immediate resection followed by colo-colonic anastomosis may be performed or, in the presence of extensive changes, a total colectomy with ileo-rectal anastomosis.

2 *In the absence of peritonitis*

Treatment should be conservative. If an ischaemic stricture should develop resection will be required, but in patients suffering from transient or evanescent colitis all that may be needed is an antispasmodic and a mild bulk laxative, a repeat barium meal being performed in order to rule out the possible development of an ischaemic stricture.

CHRONIC VISCERAL ISCHAEMIA

Chronic visceral ischaemia is a much discussed but seldom encountered pathological condition.

Aetiology

It may be associated with—

1 atherosclerosis of the coeliac, superior mesenteric or inferior mesenteric arteries;
2 extrinsic pressure on the vascular supply to the bowel by neoplasms or anatomical abnormalities, particularly in the region of the right crus of the diaphragm.

Despite the high incidence of atherosclerosis of the mesenteric vessels the syndrome of mesenteric angina is uncommon.

Clinical presentation

The commonest symptom, seen in 98 per cent of patients, is abdominal pain, often described as cramp-like, situated in the periumbilical region. It usually occurs within half an hour after eating. Weight loss is common and is found in about 66 per cent. This is partly due to starvation, which diminishes the attacks of pain, but in some individuals it is caused by malabsorption; should the latter occur the frequency of defaecation may rise to between 6 and 20 stools daily.

Abdominal examination may be negative but bruits may be heard over the aorta in about half the patients.

Investigation

1 Eliminate or confirm the presence of steatorrhoea.

2 Barium studies may show thickening of the mucosal folds, or break up of the column of barium as in other malabsorption states, usually more proximally than with other causes of malabsorption.

3 Intestinal biopsy, this may show partial or total villous atrophy.

4 Aortography: if this investigation is performed care should be taken to take lateral views of the abdomen to display the proximal parts of the coeliac axis and superior mesenteric arteries to best advantage.

Only extensive arterial disease will produce this syndrome. Approximately a sixth of all patients suffering from thoraco-abdominal aneurysms or infrarenal atheroma have completely asymptomatic isolated occlusion of the superior mesenteric artery, in which case an enlarged inferior mesenteric artery provides the collateral source of supply. Asymptomatic occlusion of the inferior mesenteric artery is also common and is particularly seen in aorto-iliac atherosclerosis and aneurysms of the abdominal aorta. However, such chronic obstruction becomes important should hypotension, from any cause, develop.

Treatment

Assuming the diagnosis is made and symptoms associated with the condition appear to warrant surgical intervention the operations of endarterectomy, bypass or reimplantation may be considered. There are, however, no large series from which the long-term results can be assessed.

4.6 DIAGNOSIS AND TREATMENT OF RAYNAUD'S PHENOMENON AND DISEASE

DISTINCTION BETWEEN RAYNAUD'S DISEASE AND RAYNAUD'S PHENOMENON

In 1862, Raynaud published a thesis in which he described the classical colour changes of the digits which we now associate with the term Raynaud's phenomenon. In the same paper he also described how symmetrical gangrene of the fingers might ensue even in the absence of organic occlusion of either the digital arteries or veins. It was this emphasis on symmetrical digitial gangrene that led to confusion. Raynaud's phenomenon includes the following features—

1 Episodic attacks during which the fingers become pallid and/or cyanosed, after which they gradually return to normal, the tips of the fingers being the last to recover.
2 Paraesthesia in the form of numbness, tingling, burning or pins-and-needles may be experienced during an attack.
3 The attacks are often precipitated by exposure to cold or by emotional upset.

The conditions producing Raynaud's phenomenon may be divided as follows—

(*a*) *Primary Raynaud's phenomenon,* not associated with any apparent predisposing cause or condition is Raynaud's disease proper. It is now accepted that the diagnosis of Raynaud's disease should remain provisional until the symptoms and signs have been present for at least two years without evidence of another causal disease.

(*b*) *Secondary Raynaud's phenomenon* is associated with contributory causes. These are many and varied and only the major groups with examples are listed below.

1 Connective tissue disorders, e.g. scleroderma, lupus erythematosus, and rheumatoid arthritis. The incidence of vascular phenomena in these three conditions is approximately 80 per cent, 25 per cent, and 10 per cent respectively.

2 Neurovascular compression, e.g. crutch pressure, the various thoracic outlet syndromes and the carpal tunnel syndrome.
3 Arterial disease, e.g. atherosclerosis.
4 Blood disorders, e.g. polycythaemia, hyperfibrinogenaemia and cryo-proteinaemia.
5 Occupational, e.g. vibrating tools, exposure to the polymerisation of vinyl.
6 Drugs, e.g. ergot, methysergide, β-adrenergic blocking agents.
7 A miscellaneous group including, causalgia, phaeochromocytoma, primary pulmonary hypertension and malignant disease.

Features of the condition that suggest secondary rather than primary disease include the following—

1 Age over 40 years.
2 Male rather than female.
3 Abnormal peripheral pulses.
4 Rapid progress of digital ischaemia.
5 Asymmetry.
6 A raised erythrocyte sedimentation rate.
7 The presence of an obvious precipitating organic disease.

CLINICAL HISTORY AND SIGNS

This is predominantly a disease of women, the sex ratio varying according to different series from 5 : 1 to 9 : 1. The common age of onset is below 40 years. Attacks beginning after this age are suggestive of a secondary factor such as atherosclerosis. The initial attacks may not be ascribed to any particular precipitating cause but as they recur it eventually becomes obvious that cold is of great importance.

The cycle of colour changes typical of Raynaud's disease is pallor, cyanosis, and redness.

Usually, the skin changes are bilateral and begin at the tips of the fingers, spreading as the disease advances to involve the whole of one or more fingers or even the entire hand. The fingers are cold during an attack and sensation is reduced, thus leading to the possibility of injury. The disease may rapidly progress until even warm weather affords little relief, or the patient may complain of perpetual coldness of the fingers even though the rest of the body is warm. Extensive gangrene is rare in Raynaud's disease, but there may be terminal ulceration and/or chronic paronychia. The diagnosis of Raynaud's disease depends on the exclusion of all known predisposing factors. This is achieved by accurate history-taking, careful clinical examination, and the use of selective special investigations.

PATHOPHYSIOLOGY

The underlying physiological disturbance in Raynaud's disease appears to be in the digital arteries and, probably, the veins as well. The initial pallor is due to spasm or obstruction which results in poor perfusion through the skin capillaries and venules. The cyanosis is due to dilated and engorged skin capillaries and venules in which the blood flow is sluggish, thus allowing time for reduction of the oxyhaemoglobin. Once the spasm is released by warming the hand the skin vessels dilate, filling with blood that passes rapidly to the skin capillaries to produce the typical red fingers.

The precise reason for the vascular constriction is unknown. Lewis, in 1922, concluded that the arterioles were hypersensitive to cold, as indeed can be illustrated. If a normal hand is cooled in water at 0°C the skin temperature falls to near that of its surroundings, but if the immersion is continued there is reflex vasodilatation that raises the temperature 5 to 8°C. This vasodilatation is short-lived but is repeated at intervals of 5 to 20 minutes. The probable benefit of this response is the possible delay of tissue damage. In Raynaud's disease this sequence is not followed. However, it cannot be the sole explanation of the vascular responses because in the disease proper the same vascular changes can be precipitated by emotional disturbance.

However, the importance of a local fault in the arterioles is also substantiated by the bad results obtained in the treatment of this disease by sympathectomy.

Blood flow through a tissue or organ is determined by the pressure gradient across the bed and the resistance to flow (Poiseuille's law). Resistance to flow is determined by the diameter of the vessel and the viscosity of the blood. The diameter of the blood vessel is extremely important because the flow varies with the fourth power of the radius, therefore, a 50 per cent reduction in the radius causes a 94 per cent reduction in the blood flow.

In secondary Raynaud's, the viscosity of the blood may well be increased by the presence of cryoproteins, polycythaemia, hyperfibrinogenaemia, or the antirheumatoid factor. The vessel diameter may be diminished in the vibrating tool groups by abnormal function of the vessel wall and the presence of microthrombi after vessel injury. In other cases of secondary Raynaud's that of the reduced flow is more obvious, e.g. atherosclerosis.

In Raynaud's disease proper, early in the course of the disease there are no organic changes, but eventually they develop. Thus, by the time amputation of a finger is necessary the digital vessels appear to have a thickened intima, and when the gangrene has occurred the digital artery may be obstructed.

DIFFERENTIAL DIAGNOSIS

The clinical history of the vascular responses together with the classical physical signs lead to almost certain diagnosis. However, acrocyanosis may be mistaken for Raynaud's. In the former condition, however, the skin changes are virtually permanent. Pallor is not usual but the hands are perpetually cyanotic and cold even in summer weather. Trophic changes or gangrene of the finger tips are never a feature of acrocyanosis despite the forbidding appearance and feel of the hands.

Investigations

The important aspect of diagnosis is the differentiation of the primary from the secondary disease. To this end, after a careful case history the following special investigations may be considered—

(a) Comb's test

This test determines the presence of incomplete antibodies in the serum which, if found, indicates the presence of an immune process.

(b) Detection of cryoglobulins

These are proteins, present in the blood, that precipitate when the serum is cooled. Cryoglobulinaemia has been described in macroglobulinaemia, a condition in which anaemia, haemorrhage from mucous membranes, generalised lymphadenopathy, hepatomegaly and splenomegaly occur. The globulin level in the serum is high and albumin low. When a drop of serum is allowed to sink in a cylinder of water a heavy precipitate of euglobulin is formed. Similar proteins also occur in multiple myelomatosis, kala-azar, malaria, systemic lupus erthematosus, and other connective tissue diseases.

(c) Immunoglobulin electrophoresis

These are present in the γ fraction and to a lesser extent the α and β. hypergammaglobulinaemia occurs whenever there is a prolonged and marked immune response, e.g. leprosy, kala-azar or chronic osteomyelitis, and also in diseases in which there is an autoimmune component such as systemic lupus erythematosus and rheumatoid arthritis.

(d) Rheumatoid factor

This is an IgM antibody found in about 75 per cent of patients with active rheumatoid disease. The antibody reacts against human IgG containing the corresponding Inu or Gm specificity.

(e) Antinuclear antibodies

These are found in about 20 per cent of patients suffering from rheumatoid arthritis.

(f) Nerve conduction studies

Should the presence of pain in the hand or the distribution of parathesiae or anaesthesia suggest the presence of the carpal tunnel syndrome the appropriate nerve conduction velocity investigations should be performed.

An abnormality in any of these results suggests a diagnosis of secondary Raynaud's.

Treatment

Relief of patients suffering from Raynaud's phenomenon consists essentially in treating the primary cause, where this is possible. Thus, the patient who develops it following the use of a pneumatic drill should be diverted, if possible, to some other occupation. In many cases, however, the primary disease is untreatable or continues to progress despite medical treatment, e.g. scleroderma. In others, some significant alleviation may follow surgery, e.g. division of the carpal tunnel when this is associated with the condition, or disobliteration of a subclavian artery injured by an accessory rib.

For the remaining patients a conservative regime should be followed for as long as possible, protecting the hands from over-exposure to cold, and keeping the body as well as the extremities warm in winter. Various preparations that appear to be of some value include, reserpine, guanethidine, griseofulvin and tolazoline hydrochloride. It has also been suggested that patients suffering from Raynaud's phenomenon due to an underlying autoimmune disease might benefit from the use of immunosuppressive agents such as azothioprine.

The object is to defer sympathectomy for as long as possible. If possible, however, this operation should be performed before the onset of actual arterial blockage. The reason for deferring surgery is the unpredictable clinical result that follows cervical sympathectomy for this condition and the known fact that at least 20 per cent of the patients relapse within a year of the operation.

In general, if the symptoms are mild, remission following sympathectomy can be expected in about half the patients whereas if the symptoms are severe only a quarter will have a long-term remission. Sympathectomy in the presence of scleroderma is practically valueless.

Technique and complication of cervical sympathectomy (see Tutorials in Surgery 1, page 305.)

Personal Notes

Personal Notes

Personal Notes

Personal Notes

Personal Notes

Personal Notes

Personal Notes

Personal Notes

Personal Notes